Men and Manners

Essays, Advice
and Considerations

David Coggins

Men and Manners

Essays, Advice and Considerations

David Coggins

Abrams Image, New York

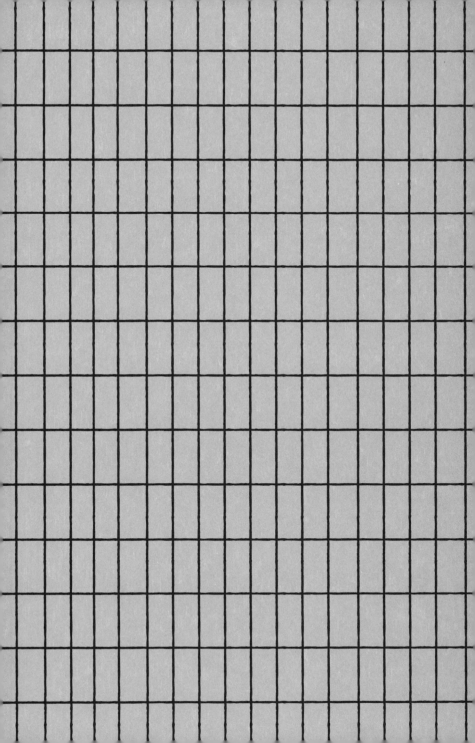

Introduction

Nobody's Perfect

I'm not here to preach. This book isn't about transporting you back to a 1950s dinner party on the Upper East Side. I'm not trying to drain your life of fun or lecture about which fork to use. The subject here is not seated dinners or when it's all right to eat sushi with your fingers (always permissible, as it happens). Manners may have once been how the upper classes recognized one of their own, about who was a knowledgeable insider and who was not. That's no longer the case.

Good manners are not relegated to town houses above the fray or for social climbers getting into country clubs. Rather, manners today are immediate and downright democratic. They're about showing fundamental decency to the people you come across every day: waiters, taxi drivers, flight attendants, strangers you meet only once.

Are certain rules helpful to know? Of course they are, and some of those enduring rules truly matter. Ideally, you'll be confident and gracious regardless of the setting, and knowing rules, and how to interpret them, puts you at ease and helps you present the best version of yourself. But some long-standing rules are really more like guidelines, and if you know them well then you know when they can be bent or even broken. But acknowledging they exist remains important—there's no civility without customs. It's easy to obsess over details, but it can be clarifying to pull back and ask one question above all: Do you try to make the lives of people around you easier?

That informs everything else. Do you give up a seat before being asked? Lend a hand? Tip well? Toast well? Listen attentively? Turn the other cheek? Make eye contact? Do you have a sense of your place in the world and your impact on others? If you have that general sensitivity then everything else falls into line. You won't conduct a phone conversation at full volume in a quiet train car. You won't prop your bare feet in public view as if you were on the beach. You won't be proudly underdressed and mistake that for a sign of authenticity. You won't text unwanted photos to a woman at 2am (or 2pm for that matter).

With everything going on in the world, it seems like a particularly good time to assess how to be a better man. Manners are now, and have always been, about making society run more smoothly. Maybe that's why there's a sense that something is missing in the culture today, that sense of civility that asks nothing in return. Too often we've convinced ourselves that to get ahead we need to take advantage of every angle. But witnessing bad behavior—in person, on television, in politics—does not excuse your own. Rather, each of us should strive to be the exception. The world may seem crazy, but that's all the more reason to be the patient, well-dressed man on the plane who doesn't throw elbows trying to get to the overhead bin.

We learn more about the world as we navigate our way through it. That's called wisdom. It's something to aspire to, and like everything worth having, it can't happen all at once. But some of the simplest rules we learned as children. And thinking of others, listening to them, basic as it sounds, is one of the animating rules of civilized life, and it endures for good reason. Manners are part of our lives whether we like it or not. Curiously, those who claim they don't care about them discover they can be quite defensive when called out.

Writing about manners is a delicate matter. Most books on the topic, as you would expect, have a certain formality. Some are out of date; others remain timeless. *Tiffany's Table*

Manners for Teenagers is worth anybody's attention at any age. Published in 1961, it imparts a sense of propriety but also a reminder that socializing, even when sitting around a table with a starched white tablecloth, is meant to be enjoyed. It recognized our humanity, including our mistakes, which is why it dealt with spilling wine and the untimely hiccup (though perhaps all hiccups are untimely). Ultimately, that book taught young people how to behave at a dinner party, and that's still a useful thing. That, however, is not the mission of this book. This book isn't about archaic rules that inspire dread but about asking more of ourselves and trying to do the better thing in real-life situations.

How did I get in this position, you ask? Who am I to judge? Did I study to be a butler? Have I even met one? Well, first of all, I don't claim to be the ultimate arbiter, eager to shake my head at some lack of decorum. But I am fascinated by behavior and dress and customs, both in America and abroad. I've written about culture, manners and the nuances of society for years. Looking back, I realize that one of my primary considerations—how men dress—is not just about clothes. It's really about being in public, how we fit into the world and how we show respect to others. Which, of course, sounds a lot like manners. All these things are connected. Which is why I'm fascinated by what people wear to the opera but also how they treat a maître d' or how they serve food at a party.

I'm confident enough to say that yes, you need a suit, and should be comfortable in one, even if you wear it only once a year. There are other things you learn through curiosity, travel and just living in the world. Manners are the guidelines of a civilized life. How you interpret those rules describes the contour of your personality. I certainly don't claim to be perfect: I've gotten in arguments with girlfriends in public (never a good look), stormed out of restaurants (also: not good). For various reasons, I've had to apologize to friends, bartenders and the CEO of the company where I worked.

In the course of my ongoing education, I've discovered that Japan is a good place to repeatedly make a fool of yourself and I've done so. It *is* possible to use the wrong chopsticks, particularly if they're for condiments that you've mistaken for an appetizer. ("This is a . . . *strong* taste.")

Yes, you tend to remember fiascos that become good stories over time. In New York I was at a black-tie affair, sat down and took what I thought was my napkin from the table. It turned out it belonged to my neighbor, a woman of a certain age who was about to be seated next to me. I realized my mistake and tried to lighten the mood by saying, "I believe this belongs to you, Madame," and theatrically presenting it to her, like a French waiter. This effort at levity was not well received. She raised an eyebrow and understandably turned away from me for the rest of dinner.

If a lot has changed since formal dinner parties, then some things have not. But technology, as a whole, has certainly altered the equation. Too easily we treat every public space as our own mobile office, catching up at full volume with friends, FaceTime-ing in the middle of restaurants, conducting meetings in outdoor voices.

So much is in flux these days, with shocking revelations of bad behavior coming out seemingly every day. Understandably a man asks himself how he fits into the world. Is it chivalrous or behind the times to pay for dinner on a first date? Who orders wine when she's the expert? Are we holding doors? Double-kissing strangers? What if they're European? We want to be sensitive, enlightened and masculine all at once.

These are questions worth asking, and I try to answer some of them in these pages. I also asked some interesting men I know what they thought about the state of play today. What does designer Todd Snyder make of the way we dress? What does the brilliant bartender Jim Meehan think of patrons on the rail? There are insights here from editors, restaurant owners, creative directors (real ones with actual jobs), behavioral scientists who've studied dating, stationers who remind you to write your mother. They tell stories, ask questions, give advice, reveal their peeves, go on an occasional rant. We're in this together, and we're trying to find out which rules still apply and which don't.

This feels like the right time to ask these questions. This is a moment when we recognize that some decency in the public sphere needs to be restored. So, in a way, I guess I am here to preach. I'm not here to call you out; I am here to appeal to your better nature. I think we know what needs to be done, so the question is how to do it with generosity and a little style.

Gentlemen: It starts with each of us. Let's ask more of ourselves as men. Let's live our lives fully; let's show respect; let's drink a martini, possibly at lunch. Let's keep our perspective, take the long view and remember that how we treat others ultimately defines ourselves. Above all, act with dignity and smile.

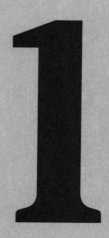

In Public

Tipping

Keep the Change

Tipping is exhausting. Not only because it's the only math most of us do. It also involves money, generosity (or lack thereof) and the possible strategic folding of twenty-dollar bills. It can signify status, it can represent somebody's livelihood, it's entwined with cultural custom, it can make somebody's day and it can start an argument. All of which is to say: it's fraught.

That's one reason we look for guidelines. Twenty percent of a restaurant bill. But what if you really went to town on the wine? You used to tip a dollar for a drink, which made sense when they were $5 but that doesn't seem right anymore now that they're $10 or even $15. You come across porters, fishing guides, room service waiters, that mercifully short-lived time when there was a separate line on the credit card slip to leave the dreaded "captain's tip" (what was *that* about?). Then you go to Europe and have to start all over again.

In Japan there's no tipping and the service is impeccable. In America we don't have that luxury and have to enter the fray, with dollar bills ready for coat check staff or men's room attendants. (I try to keep a mental list of which Manhattan restaurants still have them so I'm prepared. Men moan about this tradition, and usually they're right. But when Lorenzo Robinson—a fixture in the men's room at "21" who was an ordained Baptist minister known as the Rev—passed away, it was a sad day indeed and was rightly covered in the *New York Times*.)

Tipping is so confounding that it's been factored into the bill at forward-thinking restaurants. (In the Danny Meyer

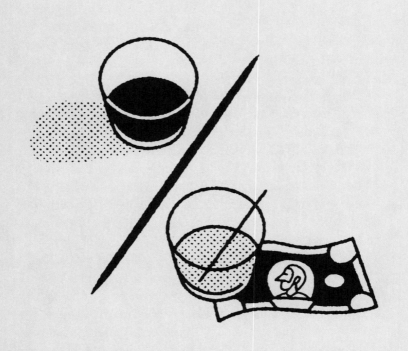

empire you can't even tip the coat check staff.) It's a huge part of the relief of riding apps where the tip is already factored in—you can just get out of the car and go.

When it comes to tipping I don't just think about the number, I think about who I'm giving money to and why. You tip because that's how somebody makes their living. You don't do it to prove something even though it certainly *communicates* something. You want to show that you are sympathetic to a bartender. Maybe a few dollars for a first drink and one for each drink after that (if it's a low-key place). If it's a more elevated setting then 20% remains a good guideline. You're not paying for just the drink but for the time you're spending there. If I'm in any setting where I sit at a table I will never tip less than five dollars (as in a diner, where the meal may be cheap).

I don't try to argue against an institutional policy by punishing an individual who has no control over it. That's to say: there may be some ridiculous service charge on your room service bill (who told you to order a burger at midnight?), but you still have to hand some bills to the server who brought it up to you. But it's also true that not every gesture deserves a tip. Just because there's a tip jar there doesn't mean it should be filled. If you've bought an embarrassingly expensive bottle of juice from a sullen teenager at a coffee shop there's no reason you have to add a few dollars to your bill.

There are occasions you don't tip—to a hotel general manager who shows you to your room, for instance. But don't get excited. There are still plenty of people in a hotel to take care of, and that will all come later—the doorman who hails you cabs, the bellboy who brings your bags, even the concierge if he's been particularly helpful. Tipping is part of the process of being in society, going to nice hotels, good restaurants, smart bars. It's the cost of doing business in an elevated way.

You don't want to tip on an already overpriced bottle of beer? Then stay at home and deepen the groove in your favorite place on the couch. I'll take the view at a good bar; you can sit, remote in hand, staring at SportsCenter highlights you've already seen a half dozen times.

If you have a bad experience then tip a little less, though it will undoubtedly be noted and sometimes asked about by a concerned manager. And that's fine. I think there's a delicate way to talk to somebody who runs a formal restaurant (not the waiter himself) if you don't like the way you were treated. If it's a worthwhile place then they'll want to know what went wrong. If it seems like they're indifferent to your plight then it's probably not somewhere you want to return to anyway.

Yes, these are the micro strategies of tipping. But in a broader sense, you want to err on the side of charity. I would go so far to say that being a good tipper is part of being a sympathetic man. You don't do it to impress, to be ostentatious. You do it because you know that a little generosity can go a long way. If you want to look at it in a purely transactional sense then, yes, if you tip a bartender you might get a free drink. But that's not why you do it.

Because cash is in shorter supply these days, you can be caught with your tipping pants down, so to speak. It's always a good idea to have small bills, but if you don't have cash when the bellboy arrives in your room, tell him you'll find him later to settle accounts. It's better just to say this directly—and of course imperative that you carry it out. It's also a reason to have an arsenal of small bills at all times. And a reminder that you're not fully dressed if you have no cash.

If you are going to a restaurant on a regular basis it's smart to be known as a good tipper; it's part of being a welcomed guest. And you can be assured that your tipping habits will be carefully noted by the staff. What kind of patron do you want to be known as? The kind who tries to give as little as possible? Or the kind who rounds up? If every diner does some benevolent math, your waitress has a good night.

If you have a relationship all year with somebody—a housekeeper, a doorman—then a year-end tip is in order. Think of it more as a gift than a tip. One hundred dollars is nice, two hundred dollars is nicer, in an envelope. (The less you pass cash hand-to-hand, the better.)

So be the man who helps a hard worker have a good day. And, as the great historian David McCullough says when advising young people (after stressing the importance of reading and having a sense of history and civic duty): leave a little cash in the hotel room for the maid. And of course, he's right. Tipping is a small bill, but it stands for something larger.

TIPPING IN BARS
On the House

Jim Meehan

Everybody loves a good bartender. Some act like you need to know the complete history of whatever cocktail you just ordered while twirling their Prohibition-era mustache. Not Jim—he's a scholar who wears his knowledge lightly. You know him from his tremendous book, *Meehan's Bartender Manual*, which may be the last such book you need to buy. (Kingsley Amis's *Everyday Drinking* is the first.) I knew I wanted a view from the other side of rail. Naturally, Jim was the first person I asked. —DC

◆ In poorly run bars with despotic bartenders, a "tip" functions like a bribe, "to insure promptness." In well-run bars with noble bartenders, a tip serves as a commission for the receipt of goods *and* goodwill.

◆ Fifteen percent is widely considered to be the minimum you'd tip—when you're disappointed with your drinks and experience—while 20% is standard for bread and circuses. Anything above 20% is considered generous by most service industry professionals. Tip no less than $1 a drink (glass of wine, bottle or draft beer, spirit pour, or simple mixed drink) and 20% for intricate cocktails and bottles of wine recommended by the server or sommelier from a list.

◆ If a bartender buys your drink or buyback (when a bartender takes food or drinks off your check as a gesture of gratitude for running up a big tab): tip a minimum of 20% of what your full check would have been if you had been charged for everything and are pleased with your drinks and service.

◆ Instead of withholding a tip following a bad experience, don't return to the bar. Your patronage and recommendation of a bar or lack thereof to others are what's at stake; not the means by which its employees earn their living.

◆ A warm thank-you made with eye contact, a wave good night or an earnest smile add gravity to your gratuity. Service professionals thrive upon the gratitude of their guests.

◆ If you pay by the round, tip by the round. If you open a tab, tip when you close the tab.

◆ Palming tips (stealthily exchanging cash by folding up a bill and shaking hands with the recipient) may be fine for bellmen and valets, but bartenders' tips should go in a tip jar—never in their pocket—so no need to be discreet. Place the tip, or signed credit card receipt, on the bar in a visible location toward the bartender's side of the counter or in the check presenter.

◆ In some countries, tipping is either not practiced or greatly reduced. If tipping makes you feel good, tip there too. You're off the hook if it's not practiced.

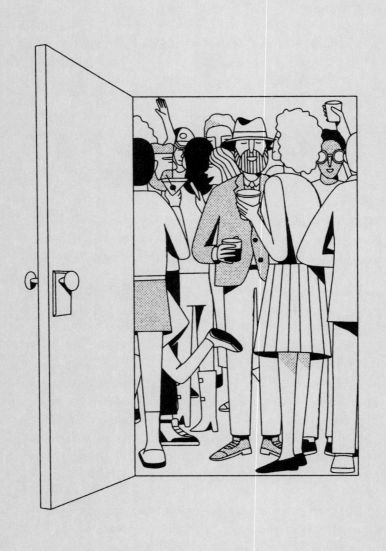

Parties

The most basic rule about parties is simple: Don't arrive empty-handed or be the last to leave. Even when your host tells you to bring nothing, still bring something. And unless you're on the cleanup committee don't be the last man standing, draining the final inch of Scotch, turning on a Smiths playlist and interpretive dancing to "This Charming Man."

You can bring wine (though not a default bottle from the store on the corner—no $8 Pinot Grigio!). White Bordeaux is an easy drinking wine. You could go into a good wine store (it's time to know one) and ask them what they recommend for a party—what I call a standing-up wine. Something people won't be too focused on, that they may not be having with food. I firmly believe in having a strong relationship with a wine store and buying by the case. It's cheaper (usually 15% off, sometimes 20%), it's more convenient, a mixed case is a great way to learn about wine, and for our purposes it's better when you're on the way to a party to take something from your collection.

Large-format bottles of wine (like a magnum) are festive, and many are not all that expensive. And they make a party more enjoyable. Of course, it's always tricky if your hosts have that type of thing sorted out. If somebody is obsessive about wine then they probably have that settled. Bring a bottle of champagne, unchilled, that they can enjoy another time. It's not for the party, it's a gift for them.

If you want to be a good guest then move around! A host loves to see you speak to an aged aunt or a shy cousin, not just the most attractive or famous person in the room. I definitely have a bad habit of staking out a corner with a trusted confidante and assessing the guests. Do not follow my lead (but if you see me, come say hello). At least greet a few people (even strangers) before locking down with your partner in crime.

I know your musical taste is the best, and that, just between us, you are a beloved DJ and really elevated some college parties. But tonight is not your night. Control the music at your own party, but defer to the host unless requested. And even then don't hijack the volume.

Of course, if you are doing the hosting then you have to prepare for a variety of factors. The first is that somebody will definitely look into your medicine cabinet "by accident" and their eye inevitably will be a judgmental one. (There is no way to look into somebody's medicine cabinet, refrigerator, closet or book or music collection and *not* make some character assessment. I remember when I was in my early twenties, before I started cooking, and my refrigerator had nothing but a bottle of champagne and a box of Chinese takeout. "Dave!" my friend said, as I was known then, "you have the refrigerator of a crack addict!") So clean that up just to be safe—like erasing your Internet history, it's just a good idea. Have the medicine cabinet as clean and minimal as a Muji catalog and rest easy. Oh, and just because you know people will be in your medicine cabinet does *not* entitle you to enter theirs. There is no innocent search for Advil.

Wiser hosts than I believe that when hosting, you want to have as much done as possible ahead of time. That way you can be out and about, not in the kitchen obsessing over details. People want to see you. And smart guests understand that they can only speak to you briefly as you have many people to entertain. (In a strange way, the better I know the host, the less I expect to speak to them. They have other people to attend to and I'm not their priority.)

Themes can be dangerous. I went to a party as a boy, in Minneapolis, where the host served Christmas cookies. There were countless shapes, enough to cover an entire dining room table. He made them all that morning and they were terrific. He also roasted a few turkeys and a ham and served everything with little Hawaiian rolls. A really simple, festive occasion. Years later I tried to do the lazy man's version of this. Just Christmas cookies, store-bought (surprisingly hard to find, and definitely a step down from my friend's). And forget the turkey and ham (my kitchen fits two people uncomfortably, sans turkeys). This was not a wild success, and I heard later that somebody begged, "We could have used something—*anything*—savory." Of course, she was right.

I believe in traditions. Once you do something twice then your friends will rightly accept it as standard practice. So have a Hanukkah party, a goth night at Halloween or a Super Bowl party (though involving the television can be risky). Anything that people can look forward to can be yours. Does your family have a recipe for rum punch? Then serve it forth! Idiosyncrasy is good. People are going to connect to what makes your party personal, not what makes it luxurious.

I'm all for aiming high or low, but in a thoughtful way. It's not about being clever, it's about your guests having a good time. And the same for when you're a guest. Be open, not contentious. If you see your nemesis consider a détente for a night. And by all means send another bottle, take your host to lunch or, at the very least, text a thank-you the next day before noon, while they're hungover and cleaning up.

Salut!

SOME HOST GIFTS
Thinking of You

To start with, I would really like to see the demise of *gift* as a verb. "He gifted me this bottle of whisky." This is one of the bad things happening in English these days (amid fierce competition). I'm not sure quite how this started, but it's really a drag. A present is given, not gifted. Something gifted sounds like a transaction between a brand and a blogger. Maybe that's why it comes off as tinny, ungracious and destined to end up next to a photo of the present on social media. Here are some ideas about things given to a host before, during and after a party or stay.

♦ Something indulgent, which your hosts will enjoy but wouldn't normally buy, is nice, like truffles from La Maison du Chocolat or smoked salmon from Russ & Daughters.

♦ If you are visiting anybody and pass a farmer's market, then get some fruit. It's of the moment, it's colorful, it feels festive. And it usually tastes great. It doesn't require any preparation; it's ready to go.

♦ If grilling is on the horizon then Newport steaks from Florence Meat Market will make you friends.

♦ Some people like the clarity of a gift certificate. I don't like seeing a price tag on a gift, and prefer to make a decision myself. An exception would be giving somebody a service (a massage at a spa, for instance, or a dinner at a nice restaurant), and just take care of the bill. That requires a little finesse and planning, but it's much more elegant.

◆ Wine from the nearest store might be a disappointment. Think a step ahead: a visit to Chambers Street Wine or Astor Wines & Spirits in Manhattan will help send you down the right path. Think beyond the default wine. My dad (who has enjoyed a few bottles in his day) recommends whites from Menetou-Salon, an area in the South of France near Sancerre.

◆ People like flowers. In fact, I don't know anybody who doesn't. They don't have to be romantic and they don't need to be for a major occasion. Like all the best host gifts, they say that you're in the spirit.

◆ Books can be a demanding gift. ("Here's something that's going to require fifteen to twenty hours of your time!") For a book that looks good and is useful, *Seven Fires: Grilling the Argentine Way*, by Francis Mallmann, is perfect for chefs, armchair chefs and anybody who's ever enjoyed a Ralph Lauren photo shoot (the gaucho Patagonia style is amazing). A book about Axel Vervoordt is ideal for an interior design obsessive—they're all nice but *Timeless Interiors* is particularly sweet.

◆ Something useful or elegant: On the subject of grilling, then a charcoal tower from Weber (the best $15 you can spend), or nice wood-handled grilling tools. A Laguiole bottle opener is a smart choice.

◆ I think it can be nice to bring (in addition to something festive) something very practical. To a party that might mean a few bottles of sparkling water; maybe good tonic, something your host might have overlooked. (I laughed at Q Tonic when it came out and I regret it: it's terrific and really lets the flavor of gin shine through.)

◆ I always like a good bottle of liquor because it lasts a while. And it can be indulgent and a variation on something your host likes. If he's a Laphroaig man, then get him a bottle of fifteen-year instead of the usual ten-year. And if he likes Scotch at all he'll probably enjoy entering the world of Rhum Agricole, the wonderful aged sipping rum from Martinique that's good in warm climates.

◆ Champagne is a foolproof gift. But try a bottle that's not one of the usual suspects. Deutz is great. André Clouet or Louis Roederer are still smart standbys. I like any blanc de blancs, which will be on the dry side, like Ruinart (which isn't hard to find) or Delamotte. And a secret of New York is that Sherry-Lehmann Wine & Spirits, the blue-chip wine merchant on Park Avenue, deals in so much champagne that their prices are usually the best in the city.

Toasting
In Good
Health

There's no toast like a bad toast. They live in infamy in the collective memory of all who witnessed them, like foreign invasions. I remember one by a father of a bride that involved moaning. A bad toast makes sense in a Will Ferrell movie, but in our lives we try to avoid them. Before they've become etched into legend, of course, we must sit through them in shared social agony.

Crying, laughing, inside jokes, swearing—all of these things move away from the simplest point of a toast: Honor the man or woman of the hour. You want to put some thought into it without the serious look of a man defending his thesis. The toast is difficult because everybody knows what you're trying to do: pay tribute, be funny, be touching. Giving a toast often requires satisfying three generations of people (if you're at a wedding), some of whom may have been drinking, and all of whom are expecting an insightful tribute to a friend that should also be concise. Oh, and have them rolling in the aisles.

There are things you can't predict. I remember being at a groom's dinner and his grandfather spoke movingly—his wife had recently died—about family and continuity and the grand scheme of things. There wasn't a dry eye in the house, and I heard a few muffled sobs that were only disrupted by an unwelcome "And now I think Dave has something to say!" This was the groom's brother, and he thrust the microphone into my hand, much to my surprise. I'd written a limerick— light verse has its place, and this clearly was not that place (it referred to the fact that the groom wore a Wellesley sweat- shirt from the bride's alma mater, a sign of true love). But since these were Minnesotans who were used to the fierce disappointment of their sports teams, I was familiar with the slightly resigned but apologetic way they gazed at me.

In other words, it's hard. But when something is hard, try to keep it simple. You can add salt to taste (so to speak). But the errors in giving a toast usually err on the side of the ribald not the chaste. Dirty stories are rarely as funny spoken aloud in mixed company as they are when whispered to a fellow conspirator. Above all, you are there as a vehicle to describe your friend. It's never been less about you than it is at that exact moment. You are there to articulate the affection that everybody has in that room for him. You do that by illuminating his character, a well-chosen eccentricity and the effect he has had on his friends and family.

It's not the time for you to roast him. If you're in doubt about sharing something then leave it out. In a perfect world, you leave guests with a clearer understanding about the man you're honoring that day. Make sure the spotlight is on the right subject. And that you get out with everybody's dignity intact.

A TOAST EQUATION

Here's How

◆ **Introduce yourself.** Never speak in public without explaining who you are and why you are there. Do this quickly, but also communicate that you're happy to be there to celebrate your friend with the people who care about him.

◆ **Explain your connection to the toastee.** Did you go to college with the groom? Get your first job from the boss who's retiring? Did you suggest the lawyer who got your uncle released on parole?

◆ **Reassure people it will be short.** When you intone, "I'd just like to say a few words about ..." make sure you mean it. Nothing makes guests more nervous than when they see you take out a ream of paper from your pocket.

◆ **Add an insightful anecdote.** You know the one—it reveals the toastee's character. Short and of course funny if possible.

◆ **Winning conclusion.** Pull it together and look for the future. If your friend is getting married, mention the bride and say this is why they're destined for happiness (in a less sentimental way, naturally).

◆ **And raise your glass at the end.** It *is* a toast, after all.

Driving Right of Way

We know you're a good driver. Better than good—you're the best. So much skill and knowledge, yet constantly being disappointed by the people around you who are, let's face it, lacking the long view you possess. It's a burden. But it's a burden you must bear because driving, for better or worse, involves navigating the shortcomings of others.

As a teenager I began a long, stormy love affair with Saabs. My dad saved an article from the paper (long before the Internet) that talked about becoming a less aggressive driver. I'm not sure I internalized it at the time, but something connected, because decades later, I still remember the major tenets. It says a lot about human nature that what made little sense to me as a teenager is eminently logical to me as an adult.

The first is this obsession (a fairly male one, to be sure) with "making good time." We proudly remember the fastest trip to the airport or some familiar landmark. Beating a round number is a real thing—making it to Cape Cod in under two hours, to the lake in three, to Vegas in four. These legendary times are passed along like statistics in an MVP season.

But, of course, you're not in the majors. If you're in the desert, the Autobahn or a closed track, then test your skill. But on the road, you're part of society and interacting with people through machines. It's always a shock just how much people become transformed behind the wheel. In traffic they behave toward others totally differently than they would face-to-face.

When you speed and aggressively weave in and out of traffic, you shave, what, a few minutes off your time? The long-ago article suggested an idea that I practice when I make the familiar drive out to our family cabin: Don't register the exact time you leave. Then you're not engaged in an arbitrary race against the clock. When you're not trying to beat your best time, you're liberated, and it makes a surprising difference.

As I get older, driving is not the real-life version of a video game I'm trying to win. As soon as you see things through that filter there's less pressure to master the road. There will always be somebody driving like an idiot, often in a red car. By all means avoid them. But it's not your duty to communicate that you think they're foolish—it's too big a job, and one that never ends. Of course it's a drag when somebody cuts into your lane at the last second. Shrug your shoulders and move on. I'll let tailgaters pass. I want them out of my rearview mirror and out of my life. It takes discipline but it's the wiser move. If you're that furious then comfort yourself with the knowledge that they may end up in hell.

It's not always easy. There are countless archetypes of drivers who are a menace (and usually in the exact car you would expect them to drive), but the road is not a courtroom and you are not a judge. I think driving is where so many of our ideas about fairness and skill and getting along come into play. That's why it makes us insane. We feel like we're the defenders of the platonic ideal, sinking in a sea of crazy, disrespectful teenagers.

I'm not in as big a rush to get everywhere, which definitely comes with age. If your wife is in labor then by all means floor it. But if not, you arrive fifteen minutes later. You're conscientious, you know how to drive a manual transmission, you don't tailgate and never honk unless somebody is about to crash into you. This was in the article too. Maybe I shouldn't be surprised that it took me that long to remember the piece. Sometimes you take the scenic route to arrive at common sense.

Plans
Make or Break

The seamlessness of technology is a blessing for making plans and a curse for breaking them. Your friend texts to say he's free and you meet at a nearby bar—love it. Or you're about to see somebody, and the weather turns bad, and you get that text in the gray area of 6pm that they can't make it—not so great. (I have a theory that this is the time when people arrive home from work and just lose the energy to head out again.) Unless of course you didn't want to go out yourself. There's a wonderfully guilty pleasure when somebody cancels on you and you secretly didn't want to see them either.

But what we really need to address is the integrity of plans, which is about respecting people and their time. I would much rather somebody be late to meet me than to be late myself. Generally I try to meet in a place where I can read or write or drink, so waiting is not bad. In fact, a friend who is a well-known writer always waits for me when I arrive. I'd come early and he would be there. I'd come radically early and he would calmly be sitting there. I found out later that he liked writing in that time when he felt the peculiar anticipation when he never knew how long he had. Good advice.

There are few good excuses to keep somebody waiting—couldn't get a cab, traffic, trains running behind; you can predict all of these things. None of them sound great but we trot them out again and again. In a sense they're code for: I didn't plan well.

Our phones make it seem like we're behaving well (texting to warn of our tardiness) when we're not. It seems that in the analog era we were more punctual—we couldn't text with our lateness notices: "There in five, sorry." Which usually means there in fifteen and not really that sorry.

Are you serially late? In a moment of extreme honesty, take a second and address this question—though that's a question that may not be something anybody can honestly assess about themself. People think they're punctual the way they think they have a good sense of humor. The way to find out is to ask your friends. Would they (secretly, of course) describe you as always late?

Or are you a serial canceler? When you enter a plan in your metaphorical book do you pencil it in (as if it lacked permanence) or is it written in ink? Not all plans are created equal—if you are going to a dinner party in somebody's home, or anywhere where there's a seat saved for you, then cancel at your social peril. When name tags are involved the canceler has nowhere to hide, as the hostess waves around a piece of paper with their name carefully written in calligraphy, saying, "Where was he *anyway*?"

There are some interesting excuses out there. "I had a work emergency" is vague, but somehow "My wife had a work emergency" is even vaguer and harder to verify. Use both sparingly. Don't start a cascade of white lies that involves keeping track of who used which excuse when. You hear somebody was under the weather and then see them waterskiing on Instagram. Don't let social media make a liar out of you. But of course who started down that road in the first place?

Broken plans are related to the sense people have of their own busyness. At this point, let's all presume we're all busy and move on from there. But we all know truly busy people and they're usually the ones who value punctuality. Which is a lesson worth learning before it's too late.

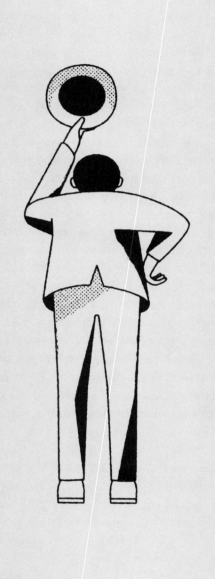

Greetings
Hail Thee Well

Greetings are the most simple custom that somehow seems to elude us. It should be simple: eye contact, firm (but not bone-crushing) handshake, slight smile. Traditionally you might say, "How do you do." My grandfather said this, as did Cary Grant, and I do too. The old-fashioned response is to answer "How do you do" right back.

But there's more than that. Hugging, half-hugging, kissing, the rest of it. It can be confusing, but remember this: Never be the first to fist-bump. That's the realm of world-class athletes and bad game show hosts. If you are not an NBA all-star then shake hands in a way your grandfather would recognize.

A greeting is a way to communicate your openness to friendship, not to exercise some power play. Nobody likes a limp handshake, but the reverse is also true, and having your fingers crushed is not how to get off on the right foot. A greeting is about measuring the moment. There is a real art to know when to move on, whether at a party or on the street. Sometimes I think the height of sophistication is when somebody you kind of know sees you on the street and says hello and just somehow understands that you both should move on.

Greetings often involve introductions. If you're talking to a friend and somebody else arrives, then introduce them right away; don't leave anybody silent and unknown. A good introduction puts everybody at ease and brings the conversation along quickly. However, if you are the person waiting to be introduced and that introduction doesn't come, then perhaps the mutual friend has forgotten a name. Jump in there and say hello, introduce yourself and save your friend embarrassment.

If we're getting down to ways I judge a restaurant or hotel, then how they greet their guests is very important. A smile and a word of welcome are indeed welcome. Somebody who simply says, "Name on the reservation?" does not belong in the service industry and signals that a restaurant or hotel doesn't have its act together.

Further, if you've stayed at a hotel or visited a nice restaurant they should welcome you back: "It's nice to see you again . . ." It's never good when the server says, "Have you dined with us before?" The answer is either, "Yes, many times, I'm sorry you don't remember," which is less than ideal, or "No, we haven't, since we're months behind the times. Please explain how the menu works, since we can't figure it out." This is the type of place that undoubtedly has shared plates and other highly detailed recommendations from Chef.

Between hotels or restaurants and guests, it's a two-way street. It's not a surprise to me that every restaurant and hotel I've loved had a great staff. You get to know them. You call them by their first name. Oh, and, naturally, you shake their hand and look them in the eyes when you arrive.

BAD EXCUSES
"You Don't Say"

If you have a real reason to miss something then be direct, say exactly why and apologize. Specificity is good, vagaries are not. That's why legitimate reasons ("I'm having an emergency root canal") inspire sympathy and understanding, and more general poppycock ("I think I'm coming down with something") does not.

A few more you don't want to hear coming out of your mouth (though when people have a bad excuse they usually text it, out of shame).

◆ "I have a work thing." (Related: "My spouse has a work thing.")

◆ "I'm really tired." (Usually followed up with, "And I've been really tired lately, a lot is going on at work.")

◆ "I'm about to leave town and have to get ready."

◆ Anything pet-related.

◆ Using the word "overwhelmed" as in "I'm just really overwhelmed with this piece I'm writing" is just a synonym for bad planning.

RECEIVED WISDOM
Lessons Learned

TIPPING

"My father was always an appropriate tipper. Not a large, showy tipper, but a sensible, 20–25% tipper. That has always stuck with me. I remember once asking why he still tipped when service was bad and he explained to me that he did so because you never know what that waiter might be going through on that day and you should have compassion. That thought remained with me, especially when I worked as a waiter." —**Jacob Gallagher**

DINING OUT

"Always reach for the check first. There's nothing more gentlemanly, in any company, than being the one to settle the bill without hesitation." —**Chris Mitchell**

PARTIES

"Always top off a guest's wineglass without being asked or asking. To ask, 'Would you like more?' is to imply a lack of self-control, if not alcoholism, on the part of the guest, and invite the inevitable, sheepish, 'Oh, really, I shouldn't,' followed by, 'No, please, really, we're all having another splash.' It's a tiresome back-and-forth that just mucks up a good dinner party. To top off without asking is really an intimate act of friendship—'It's great to see you, let's throw caution to the wind tonight'—and it's also a subtle compliment: 'I know you know how to have a good time, but I also know you are grown-up enough to know when to say when.' Guests can always leave a full glass of wine on the table if they are driving or have to catch an 8am flight the next day. But on the chance they do want to extend the evening, the last thing you want to do is leave them begging or apologizing." —**Alex Williams**

"I've definitely knocked over glasses of red wine at dinners and been mortified, but my Achilles' heel is still knowing which wineglasses are mine. I chalk it up to being left-handed, since I'm invariably reaching for a dinner companion's glass." —**Chris Mitchell**

GREETINGS

"I've always felt that asking good questions was a better form of communication than making declarations. Though perhaps that is just my way of concealing the fact that I'm not an expert in anything." —**Ben Greenberg**

"I'm a bit out of my depth with cheek-kissing. The number of kisses and order of cheeks varies throughout Europe and even within different regions of France. As pleasant as it is to kiss a Dutch girl three times, it can be hard to remember the rules. I once planted an awkward smooch full on the lips of an older woman when we each misjudged the other's initial trajectory. It's a potentially hazardous feint-and-thrust process that begs a natural talent." —**Natty Adams**

PLANS

"I always try to be on time for any sort of meeting or event. I find the phrase, 'time is money' to be a bit misleading. The way I think of it rather is that time is the one thing that we share, and it acts as an equalizer. The one thing I can be absolutely certain of is that they have a finite amount of time in a day. So I consider promptness as a sign of respect. It's a sign of good faith that I understand that you are constantly faced with this limitation and I will never value myself higher than you. So I do my best to arrive on time. It starts things off on the right foot, and frankly, he who arrives first is always most prepared! Yes, it's self-satisfying, but if I arrive first then I can pick where we sit, what I'm doing when you arrive, what my body language conveys to you as you approach. It's a control thing, but it is also a courtesy thing. How rarely do those two things align!" —**Jacob Gallagher**

GRIEVANCES
This Is Killing Me

PLANS

"The number one thing in this world (as in the social world we move in) that I despise is the offhand 'Oh, let's get a drink sometime!' comment, with *zero* follow-through, that I hear time and time again at all the work events that I attend. Or even just passing someone I casually know on the street! I don't care if you want to get a drink or not, but don't say something and then not have the chutzpah to actually send a follow-up. It feels shallow and absentminded and I find it a poor reflection on one's character. If you are saying you want to take an action, then do so. Be confident to put yourself out there, don't just give me Doppler-effect lip service as you pass me by." —**Jacob Gallagher**

"When paying for a restaurant bill, the waiter should never come back to the table with more than two leather check booklets. We have all kinds of tech to give our friends money immediately without having the physical currency in hand. Pick up the bill, tell your friends to use whatever app to pay you back. Your guests will thank you, your waiter will thank you." —**Christopher DeLorenzo**

DRIVING

"Not using turn signals. And while we're at it, same goes for not acknowledging when someone lets you over." —**Jonathan Baker**

RESTAURANTS
The House Recommends

Brooks Reitz

Some people are naturally good hosts and gifted in the art of hospitality. From the first time I met Brooks, who owns a series of restaurants in Charleston, South Carolina, I knew he was one of these men: thoughtful, generous and not too fussy. So I asked him for some advice for diners, from the restaurant's point of view. —DC

◆ Canceling a reservation within hours of your scheduled time is just plain naughty; we have a hard time recovering when we don't have time to rebook those seats.

◆ Food prices fluctuate, and good products cost money. If you're at the table, what good is complaining about the pricing?

◆ The greatest thing a customer can offer is an understanding of the promised experience. A pizzeria may not have a maître d', and a fine French restaurant may not offer PBR in the can; a reasonable customer will understand their surroundings and adjust their expectations appropriately.

◆ Open kitchen? Swing by for a quick "well done" for the team behind the stoves. Their heads may be down and engrossed in their work, but an appreciative attaboy from their customers means more than you will ever know.

◆ Is the bar fully slammed with people waiting for seats, or is it a midday lull with a relaxed vibe in the air? If it's busy, it helps to have your order on hand to ensure efficient service. If it's quiet, the barman will have more time to talk. Either way, they are happy to have you; they just might not have the time to catch up when balancing a full bar of eager patrons.

◆ Yelp has its merits, of course—but nothing will more effectively address an issue than speaking to a manager, in person and in the moment. You'll be surprised at how quick we are to make things right or to address short-comings. They happen, but we'd always love the chance to fix them quickly rather than read about them later.

◆ We welcome omissions. We loathe substitutions.

BARS
More Advice for Men on the Rail

Jim Meehan

◆ Be ready to adapt your behavior based on the type of
bar you're in. Yelling and screaming in a busy sports
bar when the home team is playing may be acceptable
or even encouraged; but it's outrageous in an intimate
restaurant or cocktail bar. Be aware and respectful of
each venue's customs and decorum.

◆ A good bartender will greet you upon arrival and serve
each guest based upon the order in which they arrived.
If you're eager to be served or engage the bartender, keep
your eyes trained on theirs, as it's the most efficient form
of communication in a busy bar. Never wave, call or get
up and follow your bartender to get their attention.

◆ Respect other patrons' personal space. If you see two or
three people sitting together, communicate to the bartender on either side of the party instead of behind them.
Be wary of those around you if you gesticulate when
you're talking and be mindful of bulky outerwear or bags
sprawling into aisles or under other guest's tables.

◆ Never name drop. If you know someone who works at a
bar (or owns it), make sure they know you're coming so
they can make arrangements in advance.

◆ Always read the menu (if there is one) and if you can't find something you'd like, have four or five classic drinks most bartenders can make in mind to request instead. Provide your server with your preferred spirit base (if you're particular) and information about how you'd like your drink to be mixed. Common preparations include ordering your martini "wet" or "dry," your whisky "neat" or "on the rocks" or your margarita with or without salt. Do not ask your bartender if any of their drinks are "sweet" or tell them you don't want a "sweet" drink. They know this.

◆ Do not feel emasculated by a drink served in a coupe or garnished with a piece of fruit or a flower instead of a hulking crystal old-fashioned glass with an iceberg in it or a steamy talismanic chalice. Any gender-related anxiety stemming from the way your drink is prepared and served belies issues your bartender is unequipped to ameliorate over the bar. Just roll with it.

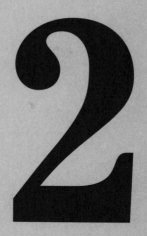

In Private

At Home
Domestic Gods

If you've ever lived with a black leather couch you should destroy all evidence of it. The male domicile that revolves around a large television where ESPN is the default channel should be abandoned in college. You are more than a sports fan or a fraternity brother. You are an individual, a thinker, and have even watched a Truffaut film on TCM. Your home should reflect that. You don't have to live in a mood board for an interior design magazine, but when people visit your apartment they will definitely take your measure by it. How you choose to live—even if it's the life of an ascetic—says as much about you as how you dress. You may choose to avoid that type of statement, but that, of course, is itself a statement.

A woman you bring home is going to judge you on your towels and sheets, probably your couch as well (and *certainly* if it's black and leather). That's certainly within her rights. If you don't think women have informed and strongly held opinions on décor then you've never been to an IKEA with one. If you bring somebody back to your home ahead of schedule you don't want to have to hurry ahead of her like an advance team before a foreign dignitary, hiding dirty laundry and throwing empty pizza boxes into the recycling bin.

There are aesthetic reasons for this, of course, but also reasons of character. How we choose to be in private says a lot about us. For starters: Let it not be in a state of sloth. There may have been a time when it was vaguely charming to have a messy room—that time is behind you.

I'm always fascinated by old photos of men in dressing gowns, which seem like the most formal way of relaxing. A big cardigan will do for me. I respond to a man who has a

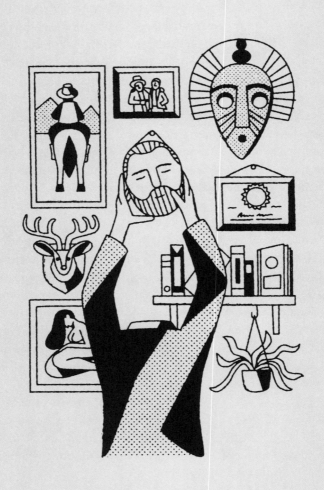

comfortable chair, maybe even a beloved blanket, and a stack of *Paris Review*s he's been meaning to read for about five years.

An art collection? Hell yes! Everything can be gifts or cost $100, but start getting artwork or photographs or pages of books that you like and put them in frames. Everybody starts somewhere. When people ask me what art to buy (I wrote about art for many years), I feel like they're forgetting that it's more than an investment. In fact, forget the investment; buy something you like to look at. Not a poster of your favorite athlete or film you adored in high school. A painting. A print. Silent auctions and fundraisers are good places to buy work. You're not going to that sort of thing? Give a little money to a good organization and see what happens.

Almost everything you do in life gets easier over time. One day you might be giving an interview to *World of Interiors* wearing a dressing gown in your winter garden. You can be telling the reporter how you used to live in Boston with four other seniors with a mini-fridge and a black leather couch. Now you're an expert in Japanese prints of the Floating World. Just look at how far you've come, baby.

Family Rules

Lessons from Above

Manners are taught to us before we know what manners are. In the beginning, they seem arbitrary and handed down from on high. This is how things are, we're told, and we promptly want to know why. Parents, out of a well-earned sense of exhaustion, reply, "Because that's just the way things are." This does nothing to satisfy the child but is understandable since the parent doesn't want to engage in a lengthy discussion of table manners or some other form of propriety. Or perhaps they just don't know, and there's nothing wrong with that. Sometimes custom has outpaced logic, and we're left wondering which glass is for wine, which for water, and why. Though what the child really wants to know is *Why can't dinner just be dessert?*

As we grow older, the world starts to make more sense. You realize that some things have logical reasons behind them. Reasons not to swear in company, arrive drunk at the office party, wear sweatpants in public at any time. But some things are just done because they've been done for a long time, like taking off your hat when you're inside.

But still this generational friction persists, and when it's not at the dinner table, it usually plays out over issues of the wardrobe. Especially when special occasions are involved. A beloved jersey is banished from a bar mitzvah. A novelty hat disallowed at Easter supper. That's partly because young people often become obsessed with an item of clothing and love and wear it intensely. The love is so intense that it does not want to be removed. When I was around six, I had a white Adidas swimsuit with three blue stripes down each side. During spring break, after a day at the beach, these trunks, which were some synthetic fabric, would dry quickly, so I felt under no compunction to remove them. This swimsuit was like the oxygen I breathed—something that felt natural everywhere I went but also was key to my survival.

As I walked down the stairs to dinner, my dad saw me and sent me right back up: "You do not wear a bathing suit to dinner." He said "you," but I think he meant humanity. One simply doesn't arrive to an indoor dinner dressed in a swimsuit. I persisted. He remained firm. "If you do that you might as well just come naked to the dinner table."

This was a blow. I knew from his tone he was beyond changing his mind. I stormed upstairs. My uncle, a musician, crooned gently, "Let's come naked the dinner table, let's all come naked to the *din-ner ta-ble*." My sister laughed hysterically. Stubborn, I changed into a towel and proceeded down to try my luck again. I was going to come *nearly* naked to the dinner table.

"*David!*" my dad fumed. I quickly beat a retreat. There are rules you don't know as a child. And it takes years to learn why the things you never understood are correct, and have been and continue to be. My sister and I still sing that song from time to time; the words we heard thirty-five years ago represent the chorus of a lesson learned.

Miscalculation
Mistakes Were Made

I went to a party at a dive bar that was celebrating its birthday. They roasted an entire pig, served good bad beer and put a lei on you when you walked in the door. *Wait, a lei?* That's just what I said, and politely declined. But then I thought, What the hell, get in the spirit of the thing. And for whatever reason, wearing a lei—even over a sportcoat—was totally liberating. I was somehow less self-conscious, even though I presumably looked ridiculous.

This was not some huge moment of enlightenment. I didn't embrace the aloha style and start dressing like Dr. Jacoby from *Twin Peaks*. But I did think about the unnecessary need for a certain propriety at all times. Or in another sense, if you don't always take yourself too seriously you're in a good position. When somebody makes a mistake in public, it's usually a human moment, and we are sympathetic to them. And if they respond with grace, even more so.

If you can handle that sort of mistake, say, when you knock over a drink, then you are in a better position to laugh at yourself in other moments as well. That's a skill that keeps on giving. There's not a man I admire who can't take a joke at his own expense. The ability to laugh at yourself can be funny, it can defuse a situation and it can be flattering (in that you're confident enough to deflate your vanity for a moment).

Because it removes the pressure from always being right, we can more easily—and gracefully—admit when we're wrong. There's no shame in asking for directions, gentlemen! (Well maybe once a decade, but still.) Admitting we don't know something is not always a sign of weakness. Ceding a little control can lead to a position of strength.

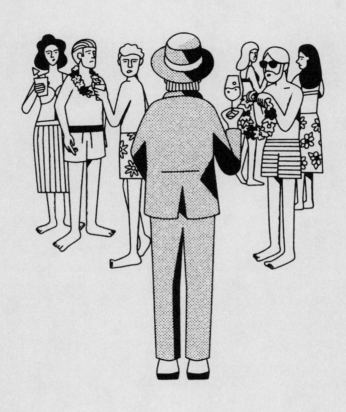

RECEIVED WISDOM
Lessons Learned

Family Meals

"When I was young, family dinner was a nightly affair.
Nothing formal, but we always set the table, closed our books,
turned down the music and sat in the same seats. Elbows
on the table? Don't even think about it. Want the mashed
potatoes? 'Would you please pass them?' And of course if it
wasn't your turn to do the dishes, you wouldn't dare leave
the table without a 'may I please be excused from . . .' My dad
didn't create these rules, but he enforced them. If my brother
and I misbehaved to a level deemed unacceptable, my father
would simply point to the door to the kitchen and we knew
what this meant. We were banished. We would have to 'sit on
the step' for the duration of dinner, which at the time seemed
like an eternity." **—Ben Greenberg**

"I can't remember exactly how old I was, but elementary-
school-aged. I was visiting my grandparents in Palm Springs
for my spring break, and one night they took me to a fancy
restaurant, I think it was called the Turf Club. I loved a fancy
dinner as a kid! After the salad course, the waiter came to
the table with an assortment of miniature sorbet cones—
that I now realize were palette cleansers—and offered me
one, which I refused. He insisted but I again refused while
informing him that 'I have dessert after dinner.'"**—Chris Benz**

GOOD MANNERS AS POETRY

Dobby Gibson

How many poets do you know? Most people don't know many, or even any. Except poets. They seem to know quite a lot. Some even play tennis together. A famous painter once told me that poets are the most competitive people he knew (and he played tennis with John McEnroe). But Dobby Gibson, a poet, writer and teacher, takes a gentler stance. I asked him what he thought of the state of manners and was not surprised he had something insightful and perceptive to say. —DC

No one ever says, "In general, I think manners are really improving!" Manners are in a terrible state of decline; this has been the assessment of everyone, everywhere, always. It would be rude of me to protest.

And yet, little flourishes of considerate social behavior still appear, usually in clusters. It's hard to imagine decorum ever fully extinguished, despite all evidence to the contrary now beamed constantly into the phones in our pockets.

With apologies to Wallace Stevens, I believe good manners are a kind of poetry.

Just as poetry too easily disappears from our daily

lives without notice, so too can manners quietly vanish or suddenly feel quaint. Then a loved one dies. Or a dear friend gets married. Or a cherished coworker announces a departure. Or a friend simply has a bad day. A moment requires carefully chosen words and the perfect gesture, and we rediscover we still have access to our more generous selves.

That's what makes unprompted politesse especially charming. Like a little work of art, the best manners serve no practical purpose and are presented with no expectation of reward. A door is held for a stranger, a handwritten note of encouragement is left on a desk, for no other reason than to prove to one another we share access to a higher form of citizenship.

Good manners can be as indelible as a great meal. Twenty years after the fact, my wife and I still recall with delight a time we were leaving a store in Umbria in a downpour. The Italian storekeeper followed us all the way to our car, holding his own umbrella over my wife's head with great care. We thanked him profusely and drove away in wonder.

The origin of my association of manners with poetry dates back to "Table Manners," a poem by the now-forgotten popular American poet Gelett Burgess, which my mother had framed and hung discreetly—or so she thought—in the kitchen of the house in which I grew up. To this day, forty years later, my sister or I will recite this poem, always loudly and in a cartoonish, Jon Lovitz–style

British accent, making sure we're within earshot of our dear mother (who has impeccable manners, naturally).

The first stanza goes:
The Goops they lick their fingers,
And the Goops they lick their knives;
They spill their broth on the tablecloth—
Oh, they lead disgusting lives!

Hysterical laughter follows, and then a hug and a kiss for Mom. (Teasing is the sincerest display of affection in our family.)

Like all truly dreadful poems, "Table Manners" has an axe to grind. And yet, when my family is done laughing, and later done dining together, we all place our silverware on our plates at precisely three o'clock, without thinking twice, to make it easier for one another to clear the plates from the table.

Gelett Burgess will always have the last laugh. Too bad he's no longer alive. I clearly owe him a handwritten note of gratitude.

FATHERS & FRENCH COOKING

A Conversation on Food with Hugues de Pins

A chef who's skilled and easygoing is something I admire. It's hard to cook well for others and even harder to keep the tranquil vibrations going. It seems French people are really good at this, because of course they are good at it. I was sitting with Hugues on his terrace as he grilled a rack of lamb and didn't really seem to be paying much attention to it. He served it with some grilled vegetables and a simple green salad, and it was perfect. I wanted to hear what he learned from his very French family about cooking, manners and inheritance. —DC

Was there something specific your father taught you?
I think what makes my dad very special to me, and to other people who know him, is that he's an excellent cook. I learned from him how to cook but, more important, the passion of cooking for others. What I learned is how much care, how many details, how much time he'd spend to prepare a meal for his family, his friends, which for me is really perhaps the most beautiful thing in life: to prepare a nice meal for the people you love. My father comes from an old French aristocratic family, and you would never see a man cooking or even standing in the kitchen. He was probably the first in his family and in his generation of friends to break the mold and to spend

hours during weekends and evenings, just to cook for the others. That was the best lesson I ever got from him.

When you were a boy, did you realize that that was special, or did it occur to you as you got older that he was the first in his generation to do that?
I think it came later. I knew it was his passion; he wanted to be a professional cook, and his father told him, "No, no—you'll do what every other man in the family has done: You'll be an engineer, so you'll go to engineering school and maybe if you like to cook you can cook at home." Which he did. It was a passion at first, and what I liked is that he converted this passion to something bigger, something he could share. But as a kid, I was not even allowed in the kitchen because he was so meticulous, he wouldn't allow us to touch anything or taste anything. It was—it still is—a religious thing for him.

When you got to a certain age, did he ever teach you something in the kitchen?
No, never. He was not really much into transmission. It was more something solitary. It was more leading by behavior. When I moved into my own flat I was enjoying cooking by myself. And now my kids love to cook as well. It was a whole cooking tradition, which started with him.

I'm always curious about the balance when someone is a good chef and also entertaining. When is enough? Do they have enough confidence that not everything has to

take so much refinement? Sometimes something basic is really great. Like a terrific steak, but with a simple green salad. How at certain restaurants they just put out a simple bowl of fruit at the end. It's just perfect.

Exactly. I think for me, the perfect meal is when you have those highs and lows. Too many highs is going to be too stuffy; you need to surprise your guests, and sometimes it's with just the simplest cheese or a salad. Personally, I prefer to put the emphasis on the products, the ingredients.

We can just pull back now—it's 2017 and you're in Europe or you're in New York—what do you notice about manners and about the men you meet?

So I think good manners in general are always in the first relationship you establish with someone. Yes, you can hold the door; yes, you can have the lady come into the room first—these are basics, and these are not necessarily difficult to learn and to practice and to act on. But I think what's more difficult is on the day-to-day basis, to be truly paying attention to others. This comes back to my grandfather's motto: Really make others feel important.

Do you have something that you like to serve that works well?

Typically, if it's something I can prepare in advance because I won't necessarily have the time to do this last-minute. I love to do things like chicken with morel sauce, with the base of the sauce a yellow wine from Jura, which blends extremely well with morels. That's a very traditional, more winter or fall kind of dish. But it's very, very good.

If I have more time, for instance, to do something more in the minute, I would come off for fish. I really like to have any kind of fish, usually a white fish, just simply grilled with a little bit of olive oil, herbs, thin-cut vegetables, and you can do it either in the oven with the grill or *en papillote*. It's very healthy and very easy.

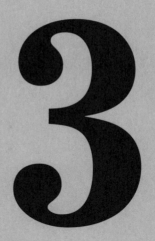

Dressed Up

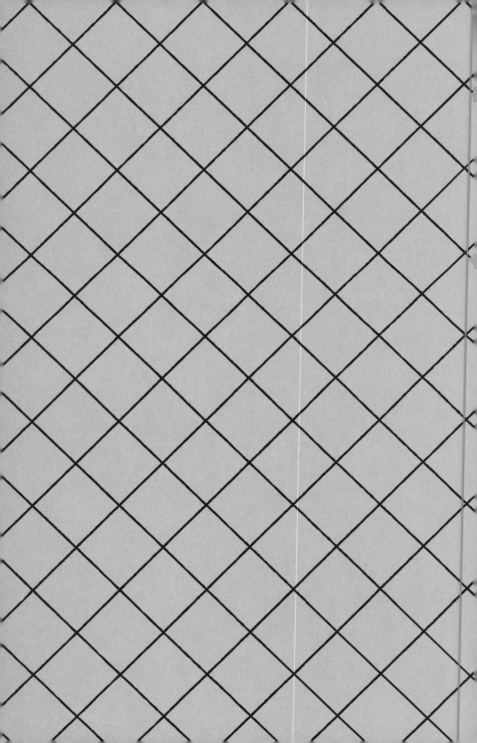

Dress Codes
Attention Must Be Paid

There are many ways to make an entrance at a good restaurant, the opera or a smart party, and being underdressed is one of the least desirable. You don't have to be a dandy, but the way you dress for an event is a matter of interest to your host, your date and anybody who is going to have an opinion about you. It's not hard to wear a sportcoat (blue and unstructured, if you want a starting point), and you should find an equation that makes sense for your figure, your salary and your position in life.

Have you decided that you are going to wear nothing but a hooded sweatshirt to indicate that you supposedly care about more important things? It's curious that in certain quarters looking slovenly has become a sign of being authentic. That's too convenient by half and not at all true. Many great business minds dress beautifully. But more than that: Who benefits when you look like you're still a teenager?

On a basic level, there's a way to show a sense of occasion and respect for the people who go out with you. If you arrive at a party, does your hostess want to see a man who looks like he just came from college after pulling an all-nighter? And if you're arriving with a woman, does she want to stand beside a man who looks like he's worn a sportcoat reluctantly, like a petulant boy dressed by his mother?

Have a suit that you feel comfortable in. Even if you wear it only a few times a year, those times are surely important. How you dress says plenty about you, but it says just as much about what you think about the people you're with. So when you stride into a room try to capture the spirit of self-expression, a sense of occasion, and you'll even flatter yourself. It's worth it.

The Sportcoat Business Partner

Let's take a moment to praise that sartorial war-horse: the blue sportcoat. If you want one thing in your closet to wear to make a good impression then get a blue, unstructured sportcoat. Boglioli makes a good one, as does Drake's. You can always get one at Ralph Lauren. If you're ever in Italy or London it seems like they sell them on every corner. One day we can talk about tweed, herringbone, double-breasted and the rest. But this is your first jacket, your counted on friend. Like your go-to whisky, it can be counted on in every occasion.

Wear it with an oxford shirt (feel free to keep the collar buttons undone). Wear it with a dress shirt and a tie and gray flannel trousers. Wear it with dark jeans, a polo shirt and R. M. Williams "Gardener" boots. This jacket should be in good shape, ready to go at any time. You don't want it to look like it survives, ill-fitting and unloved, in deep hibernation at the back of your closet. Or that your mother bought it for you against your will while you still lived at home. In many ways, this stands for your evolution into a man who's ready for whatever the day, or night, brings.

I'm not trying to make you dress in a Savile Row suit or worship at the altar of Neapolitan tailoring (though those are worthwhile endeavors). Dressing well involves self-knowledge and an understanding of how you fit into the world. Formality is not for everybody. If you follow your own path, you might be lucky enough to have arrived at your own uniform, which can be liberating despite its strictures.

On the other end is the sartorial experimentalist. I know a particularly well-dressed man who is proud to have never worn the combination of his clothes twice. That's remarkable and should be left to the professionals and the obsessives (he's both). For everybody else, there's a point when you realize what you need for your professional life and personal life. Are you committed to jeans made with Japanese denim that has a documented pedigree? Great. Do you save up for Alden boots? Well done. I love seeing men who have something nice and wear the hell out of it. Invest, keep, repair!

The first suit I got in New York at the tender age of twenty-three was a gray flannel Ermenegildo Zegna made-to-measure suit, a birthday present from my parents. I wore that thing hundreds of times. I loved it. I had to have the inner thighs of the trousers resewn anually. (This happens to suits, especially with heavier fabrics, which is why Savile Row firms used to make second pairs of trousers for their clients.) Finally, the fabric was so worn down, I vowed this would be the last repair. I brought it to a Russian tailor near my West Village apartment. There was an older man with a strong accent who worked there who seemed like he could have been a professor or some public intellectual before he moved to America. It felt like he had a heavy sense of history and sweet sadness to him. I put the trousers on the counter, sighed and said, "This is it. This is the last time I'm getting these repaired. The fabric has almost worn through." He looked at them. Anybody else would have retired these pants long ago. He looked at me. "I understand," he said almost wistfully. "You have a hard time saying goodbye." Yes! I do.

So please get those shoes resoled, patch the elbows of your tweed jacket and wear your clothes deep into their thriving middle age. Make people associate you with a great jacket, a hat, even a cologne. Yes, when your life, livelihood and sense of style align, it's a powerful place to be. And please, please let that uniform aim higher than a hoodie.

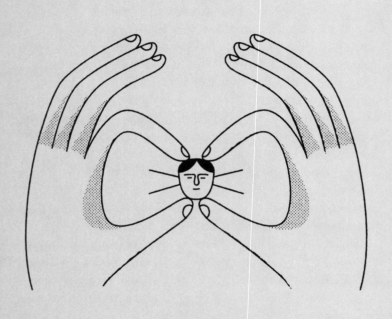

Black Tie

Like being audited, an invitation that clearly states BLACK TIE can inspire a sense of dread in the hearts of men. Of course, if you're Jack Donaghy then it's just another weekday night. But most men chafe at the thought of squeezing into a tuxedo. Why is this? Does it recall the traumas of prom night, when a group of men looking like a deposed boy band piled into a limousine with their infinitely more sophisticated dates?

Do tuxedos connote the indignities of renting a suit of clothes that have been worn by countless other men? Possibly. Is it conformity—the idea (wildly untrue) that all men in tuxedos look alike? Is it the notion, in certain corners, that to dress up is not aligned with having a good time?

Perhaps it's all of these things. But let's be clear: Men look good in tuxedos. But for anybody to look good they need a sense of comfort and proportion. That's not going to happen in a rental. There are few hard rules in this book—but not renting a tuxedo is about as close to etched in stone as you can get. (While we're at it: A true martini is made with gin, not too dry, stirred impossibly cold in a small glass and served with a twist of lemon. I thought I would sneak that in.)

When you've arrived at that stage in life, then buy a tuxedo. There are good options up and down the financial scale. Talk to the great lads at Sid Mashburn in Atlanta. Go to Ralph Lauren, go to a tailor. I prefer a peaked-lapel one button (or a double-breasted, if you're ambitious). A tuxedo should look formal, not like a black suit in disguise. You wear it only rarely? Well then you know that each time is important. A wedding, a gala, opening night at the opera. These are occasions, and you want to communicate that you understand that.

When an invitation offers some sort of variation on the classic formula—the dreaded "Creative Black Tie"—you are within your rights to ignore it and wear a tuxedo as you normally would. In fact, you should do this to remind your host that the traditional equation can't be improved upon. If you have something you've been dying to try, adding the slightest hint of color in your pocket square, for instance, then now is the time. But the same way a martini doesn't improve with novelty, a tuxedo doesn't either. If you think you've hacked the code and discovered a new idea that a century of men have missed, think again, call for help. Do anything to keep from looking like the extremely foolish Oscars attendees (there are countless every year), who try to buck the system and end up just reinforcing it.

If you don't think men are flattered in a tuxedo then look at photos of any American icon: Bogart, Newman, Astaire, McQueen, Sinatra. Black tie, served neat, flatters any man. To fear black tie is to fear being classy.

A man who owns a tuxedo is confident when an invitation arrives. He is ready for the challenge. He knows that he can drink champagne or bad beer, make a toast or push his chips in and bet it all on black. He's the man of the hour, any hour of the night and day.

Informal Leisure with Dignity

There's been a proliferation of the unwelcome view that if you dress in a sloppy way then you are somehow more authentic. This exists the closer you get to Silicon Valley and is meant to convey that you have more important matters to think about than dressing well. All it implies, in fact, is that you are authentically sloppy.

Does not having good table manners make you more authentic? Does not bathing make you most authentic of all? Of course not. You chew with your mouth closed, shower every day and never wear a hoodie to work. In any case, moving up in the world is a chance to expand your sartorial horizons. This does not mean you have to shed a uniform. Go to a tailor and tell him you'd like his finest blue suit (they're not all created equal!) or that you're looking for a white shirt meant to be worn sans tie (the stiffness and shape of the collar is different on a shirt that is buttoned up all the way and one that is not). See how easy that is?

A sense of what's appropriate extends into what you carry. Which is to say: Do you need to bring a coffee cup every place you go? There is a streak in American culture about doing everything at once. You don't stop to take a coffee (as you would in Naples, Paris or countless other cities). Here, of course, we take it with us. That ship has sailed, and there's no going back. Do you need to bring an enormous water bottle into every meeting? This fear people have of being dehydrated is a curious national characteristic. Do what you have to do. But for goodness' sake, don't bring your coffee into a restaurant. They serve coffee! That's what they do. It would be like going into a men's store to try on your own clothes in front of their three-way mirror.

When you dress well you show respect to society at large. You are not treating the fine streets of great cities as if they were the halls in a locker room. I gather you like to exercise—that's fine. But your workout clothes belong in the gym. They do not belong on the way to the gym. They do not belong on the way back from the gym. You may disagree with this in principle, but remember, as you set off down the street in sweatpants, that you might run into your ex-girlfriend, your future girlfriend, your potential employer. Or journalist Gay Talese, a man so formal, he scolded me for not wearing a suit-coat in my official author photo—a tie was not enough.

Any fabric that has a trademark or a name that ends in the letter X does not belong in a place where people are not sweating. I once saw an editor heading into his company's headquarters in an overcoat with a canvas racquet bag over his shoulder. He looked immaculate—the bag was the only sign of where he'd come from. That's as it should be.

These things are related because we are losing our connection to occasions. Instead of asking what's appropriate to wear to work, we ask what we're in the mood for. I'm certainly not a corporate type, but when I went to an office for the year I worked in one I dressed in a tie every day. But I also insisted that I not eat at my desk. That seemed like a good stand on principle. I wanted to spend an hour outside, to read the paper or sit in the park. Perhaps I'm not made for this time—but I believe a well-dressed man is still a welcome sight to the eyes of men and women alike. Put on a jacket, look smarter than you have to. Start your own corporate culture that looks good when it goes public.

Grooming
Growth
Strategy

Look at a photograph of a man, and his haircut, sideburns and approach to beardliness reveals a lot. His hair can tell you whether he's a metal musician, a cult leader or a Republican. It can tell you his era, his prerogatives or whether he ignored advice from loved ones. There are no indifferent beards or sideburns. They help you change or discover your identity, which is why young men in particular experiment with them. Some of those experiments are best left in the past, which is why men of my generation are glad Facebook didn't exist when we were in high school and traces of bad goatees could be mercifully wiped from the record.

I would be curious to meet a man who has had the same haircut his whole life. Did he come into this world fully formed? Did his musical tastes not change either? There were highs and lows in high school for me, like everyone else. I'm not ashamed of the sideburns I wore in 1991 as a Morrissey devotee. The same way his music made sense all of a sudden, so did my sideburns arrive, seemingly in an instant. When I started to shape them into the art school version of muttonchops, that was a little severe. There was a more major misstep, a mercifully short-lived flirtation with a goatee. Sometimes I think young men grow goatees just to prove they can. Sadly many young men suffer through this goateed gap in self-awareness—I think my mind was impacted by a Miami Dolphins hat I wore.

But you grow older and, hopefully, wise enough that you take a certain care in your presentation. As a man with a beard I fully support having it trimmed by a professional. A barber sees the big picture, or at least your face in three dimensions, which, of course, a mirror does not allow you to do. (If you're just taking it down with clippers, that's another matter; then you can trust your own hand.) The point is that you owe it to yourself to look like you've looked in a mirror, if only once a day.

I'm not sure where we conflated messiness with authenticity (a dangerous word in any case). There's certainly a time to be less kempt, but that time was when you were declaring your major. Now you've graduated in every sense of the word. That means higher expectations for yourself. Or think of it another way: Do you want to be held to a low standard? Far better to set the standard.

Do you remember the cologne your grandfather used? Chances are you do. On his way to becoming distinguished, he chose his scent, didn't make a fuss about it and kept a clean sheet, so to speak. Well, now's your chance. Cologne can be your friend (try one that's been around awhile and doesn't advertise in sports magazines). And if somebody you find attractive gets close to you, who knows? They might enjoy detecting a discrete scent of cologne.

I've had a beard for so long that I can't remember buying razor blades. But that doesn't mean that beards should be left to their own devices like swaths of greenery in the tropics. A beard needs to be maintained, man! You don't want to look like you're starting a religious sect—you want to look like you're upholding the noble tradition of Civil War generals, Russian novelists and French painters. Great men grew beards that suited them. Don't let your barber get too aggressive. Remember that there are no straight lines in nature, and your beard should end at your neck in a fade, not a stark line. I've left my beard untended for too long. On the quest to show solidarity with Melville while fly-fishing in Montana, I instead looked more like the Unabomber. Don't let this fate befall you!

Similarly, if you decide to go down the path of stubble, it should look like you intended the look, not like you forgot to shave. It's never ideal when a man has a slightly dazed appearance where you can't tell if he took the day off work or his girlfriend left town and he stayed up all night binge-watching old episodes of *Deadwood*.

There are extraordinary men's apothecaries in Milan, London and Paris that have been there for more than a hundred years. Why is that? Because there are things men have needed for a long time. You can be part of that tradition too— as long as you don't use body spray. If you're gay or straight, single or attached, your mother, who knows you better than most, will always appreciate when you put your best face forward. You don't want to look like the world happened to you. Take some initiative, show some intention, get your mane under control. Then, and only then, can you conquer.

RECEIVED WISDOM
Lessons Learned

DRESSING

"My father was meticulous about his shoes; it was what he lived by and still does. Whether imported, custom, dress or his old standby Florsheims, they never looked unpolished or scuffed.

"The fit was perfection, and he drove people crazy for that half-size difference. He's a mechanical engineer and a Virgo—striving for the best is part of the process. He had the shoe polish wooden box and would work on them in the back hallway. Post-polish lineups were a regular visual for me. I admire that respectful, obsessive trait and it lives on in me."
—Michael Maccari

"My father was not the kind of man to care too much about the etiquette of clothes. He never explained which occasions required a blazer and which required a sportcoat. For him, a man's presentation was less about how he dressed and more about how he spoke. To have poor grammar—to be inarticulate—was a social calamity. Greatly disturbing to him was the common confusion between the proper use of 'well' and 'good.' The correct usage of the two was hammered into me from an early age." **—Matteo Mobilio**

"My main guideline on dressing is to put some thought into it and try to be your own man. Take inspiration from everywhere you can—not just people but nature, literature and history—but never simply imitate. And dress with the aim of joy and pleasure." **—Natty Adams**

GRIEVANCES
This Is Killing Me

DRESSING

"Everywhere with the sandals. Sandals in the city. Sandals in the office. Sandals on the plane (the most egregious violation, for some reason). My dad taught me, 'Outside the house, a man should never show his toes unless there's a swimmable body of water nearby.'" —**Curt Benham**

"The reluctance of American men to wear a sportcoat or blazer annoys me. I'm a huge fan of evolving dress codes— I wear classic sneakers with suits regularly—but a jacket is something men should generally include in their dress. Going to dinner, getting on a plane, walking around a city on vacation: Put on a jacket. It's always better to err on the side of looking a little more polished than a little too casual, and good tailoring should be the most comfortable thing you wear." —**Chris Mitchell**

"Wearing exercise clothes in a non-exercise environment." —**Jonathan Baker**

NO SQUARE-TOED SHOES

A Conversation with Todd Snyder

Todd Snyder makes the hard things look easy. He's well-dressed, well-liked and successful, which is a pretty good formulation. He's low-key about clothes, despite having his own renowned line. Perhaps that's because he's from Iowa, which keeps him level-headed. I wanted to talk to him about how men dress today. Though there are good Todd Snyder suits, he's not too formal, and I knew he would have some straight-ahead advice for the men of today. —DC

Did your father teach you anything about dressing? Did he suggest any rules that you still follow?
I remember he would always tell me, "Dressing well is a sign of respect for wherever you're going." For someone's party, an event, a business meeting, whatever it is. That's always stuck with me. You show up to a business meeting and you come in a tie and a jacket, it's for the person on the other side of the table.

What questions do men typically ask you about dressing?
The rules. They always think that there are rules. What do I wear with this? There are certain rules you need to follow, but you need to know the situation, you need to know the event, and then you can make tweaks here and there. And I think that's where most men get confused.

Do you have any rules that apply to most situations?
I always default to better be overdressed than not.

Has that ever happened to you?
It still haunts me from when I was in grade school. I remember we were getting ready for some school presentation where we were all up onstage and everybody was talking about what they're going to wear. And I remember that I had only one pair of jeans that didn't have holes in them. So I didn't go to the presentation because I was so afraid of not looking good because I didn't have any nice clothes. That's the one thing that stuck with me. It's the reason I'm in fashion! I still have occasional nightmares where I wake up and I'm not properly dressed or I'm completely naked and I don't know what to do.

What are things that you notice when you meet a man?
I notice everything. I'm not judgmental. I grew up in Iowa, as you know, and now being close to fifty you kind of get perspective. You live through it enough and you see people come and go and you realize it's not that big of a deal. But I do like stylish people, both men and women. I'm always looking at everyone and that's how I get inspiration.

What are the rules? I'm not the author of the rules, I just see what the public is wearing, and then I twist it ever so slightly to make sure that it fits within those general rules. Before I go to any event, I always Google it to see what people are wearing. I went to a polo match—and what do you wear to a polo match? I still want to be myself, I don't want to show up and be somebody who I'm not. I think there's a way to do that and still be yourself, whatever event you're at.

Is there something that grieves you or peeves you about men and dressing today?
I wish men would pay more attention. I still say it—but I still see it—so I keep saying "No f-ing squared-toed shoes!" I said that one time in an event that I was at in Iowa of all places, and some guy came up and he had an amazing pair of monk-strap shoes and they were slightly—they weren't necessarily squared, but he was freaked out. Are these all right? I said, No, you're fine. They looked like some amazing pair of John Lobb shoes.

It's not hard to dress well; just pay attention. But square-toed shoes and the date shirt are my two biggest peeves.

Like a party shirt?
Right. Big collar with contrast under the collar, you flip the cuffs up, you wear it untucked. You know it. I've heard it called everything from the date shirt to the fuck-me shirt to whatever.

I can almost imagine the cologne that would go with that.
You can picture the guy who wears this, and you don't want to be that guy.

THE VIEW FROM SWEDEN

Olof Nithenius

I have never met Olof. He's part of the European sartorial firmament and he works with what must be the best Swedish magazine with an Italian name, *Plaza Uomo*. I enjoy his sensibility and was curious about what he had to say about current rules of dress. The fact that he's from a Scandinavian country made me even more curious since some sense of community still prevails there. —DC

Behavior, rules and etiquette are interesting topics I've spent some time reflecting on. The reason is that I live in Sweden, which is in some ways a very inconsistent country. Everything started in 1967, when a general-director for a state office decided that titles were not to be used in his business—everyone should call on another by their first name. This was controversial at the time but led very quickly to a less formal attitude in the society at large. Just a few years later it was no longer socially accepted to use formal titles in the workplace. It might have been the era, the political climate or reform, where the old and conservative were considered to be outdated. But for me this is still very strange. I prefer to use a formal approach in some situations—just out of respect.

I would never call myself conservative or old-fashioned. It's just who I am and how I was brought up. My parents raised me in a liberal and classical way. We were encouraged to think freely but to be correct in every situation. My mother had some basic rules, such as eat properly at the table, never wear a hat inside, never use bad language and be kind to everyone. This included respect for other people, and for me that might include a formal address.

I have been bawled out a couple of times when I have used the tram and offered my seat to older people when all other seats have been taken. What has always been obvious for me can in some illogical way offend people. And that is Sweden in a nutshell.

One thing that bothers me today is that the term *gentleman* is overused. Today many people use *gentleman* as a term for someone who dresses classically well. For me, that's very wrong. Just listen to the word *gentleman*: it's a compound for a gentle man. For me the meaning of *gentle* is far more important than being well-dressed. It doesn't matter how sharply dressed a man is if he's a bully. That being said, I can still call a less well-dressed person with a true and warm heart and good manners a gentleman. My father is a good example. He is nowadays a poor dresser, but he acts correctly and is kind in heart and soul. He treats all persons no matter of background, race, gender or age with the same respect.

For many years, he dressed in a classic and formal way. At the end of his career he dressed more casually and didn't care as much as before. I once asked him why, and his answer was that he didn't have to dress up to impress anymore. He had reached a situation where people knew what he was capable of anyway. But I deeply admire the few men out there who have a gentle and humble manner and correct behavior as well as a well-cut bespoke suit. That's something to look up to. Rules should never be used in order to make people feel uncomfortable; quite the opposite. The reason why we have dress codes is that everyone should know what to wear and what's expected. When that is achieved, everything else will be much easier.

Therefore, I prefer dress codes in formal situations such as in some businesses, and for weddings, dinners and funerals. Old and boring "rules" such as "No Brown in Town" make me laugh. I almost always wear brown shoes in town! Why? Simply because black is not a color, it's a state of mind, and there's less life in the black color than a nice polished brown. Not to mention a brown suede.

As when it comes to the use of the term *gentleman*, I think that we use the term *style* way too often nowadays. Style is for me so much more than how we dress and look. I would like to use *style* as contrary to *fashion*. Fashion for me is short-term; it's shallow and changes all the time. Style is something personal and long-lasting. A person's style should be a reflection of his personality. I respect and admire those who have a personal style and taste and don't just follow the stream. There are too many dead fish who just float down the stream, anyway.

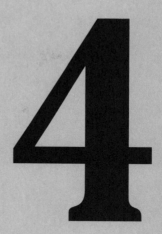

Technology

Writing Correspondence Course

I'm embarrassed to think how long it's been since I've scrivened a hand-written letter. Long emails that are actually personal: yes. Text threads with close friends and family that I guard zealously: yes, indeed. We lament the demise of writing in ink, but it's also true that we are surrounded with written communication. At work, with friends, live chat with the telephone operator. Flurries of typed words are part of modern life.

It's interesting that there doesn't seem to be much consensus on the form these should take. A busy friend of mine said nothing bothered him more than receiving an email that just said "Thank you." I finally started using exclamation points after a lifetime aversion. Now if my mom texts me "Ok," it feels oddly mercurial, possibly even hostile. "Let's get in spirit, Mom!"

Everybody thinks they're busy. You may know somebody who's truly busy and decide somebody else is not, but that person still feels like their life is on the brink of overwhelming them. All of which is to say, much of email and text is about respecting other people's time. If somebody is not vital to the conversation get them off the text thread. We are haunted by unread messages, phone vibrations, endless notifications. I get nervous seeing friends' phones with thousands of unread messages. Those red numbers are menacing reminders of an inefficient life.

For one year I unsubscribed from every mass email I received. Every one. From Belgian art galleries, English shoemakers, Tribeca theater groups, Charleston restaurants. It was clarifying. I wanted to get to a point where every email I received was addressed to me by a person I knew. That day will never come, but it was a good exercise. It helped me focus on each message—communication with purpose, directly between people.

Maybe that's why I dislike Facebook invitations. They feel so impersonal. Of course it's convenient in some way. But it also quantifies behavior in a way that seems clinical. Are you attending? "Yes," "No" and "Maybe" just don't capture the range of social options, especially if they're public.

Work emails want to be short and during business hours. Try not to email your assistant on the weekend at all (make sure your level of an "emergency" really reaches that threshold). Funny videos may not be as funny as you think and certainly should go to a small group of friends who've shared that sort of thing before. You'll want to find out what the text and email habits are of any new addition to your life, whether it's your boss or girlfriend.

Communication evolves. Now it feels strange to call somebody without texting them first to make sure they're free and to give them a warning. Phone calls are for emergencies. My sister called me a few times not long ago. I was frantic. "Is everything all right?" I nearly yelled. "Oh it's fine." "Then why didn't you just text?!" She just wanted to talk. The nerve!

There was a time—not that long ago—when people wrote long, formal emails like letters. Then there was a time when people wanted one line only, in the subject line of the email. It will continue to change as our relationship with technology changes. There will always be questions, but we can all agree that now and in the future there's no place for a text that is only "?"

Texting
Word to the Wise

Such a useful tool is the text. Immediate, brief and as personal or impersonal as you want it to be. For those of us who dislike the telephone, it's a blessing. But like all technology in its infancy, there's just an emerging consensus about text etiquette (though we can all agree that "read" notifications are deeply unsettling and perhaps even a psychological power play).

It's strange when you get an emoji from some sober-minded person. Or a LOLZ when you don't expect it. Not unlike seeing a pastor wearing red socks. My texting would be greatly improved by italics—reread J. D. Salinger to see just how useful they can be. We're talking about emphasis here. After fifteen years of writing without using a single exclamation point, my texts now abound with them. They've migrated over to my prose as well (which you may have noticed). It's gotten to the point where if my mom (a late-comer to all technology—she has her car radio set to classi-cal public radio and doesn't change it until she gets a new car) sends me a text that just says "fine," then I'm worried something is wrong. It should be "Yes, let's have lunch!"

It turns out I was upsetting some friends who didn't appreciate the bone-dry humor in my texts and took them personally. In went the emoji! (Though oddly they don't have a range of bearded men—scandal!)

My feeling about texts is that they should be short, clear, hopefully funny and, crucially, welcome. Texts work better, naturally, the better you know somebody. Though of course they can help you get to know somebody. It's no surprise that texts are used as a romantic tool. They're about

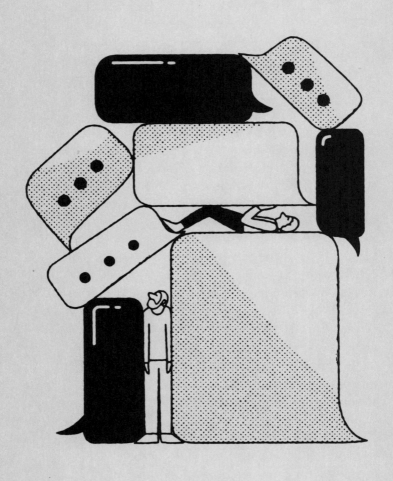

communication, imagination and also waiting. But better that some things be left to the imagination.

Since many people grew up with this technology and I did not, I won't pretend to understand Snapchat and the rest. But I do think, regardless of age, that you shouldn't be sending unsolicited and unwelcome pictures at three in the morning. I'm shocked hearing from young women how often this happens to them. I'd like to think that if men knew how often this happened to women then it would dissuade them. Don't be so predictable. I'm afraid after a certain point it becomes common practice.

I may not understand the technology but I think that some things have proven the test of time, which is that when it comes to undressing, it's good to have something to look forward to without all the secrets told ahead of time. Your au naturale photo may be the ultimate spoiler alert.

Punctuation

Word One

I'm not sure if my spelling is actually getting worse as I get older or if I take for granted spell-check riding to the rescue. While it's true that many writers have not been good spellers, I think most of them take their punctuation very seriously. It doesn't rise to the same level as Martin Scorsese threatening to take his name off of *Raging Bull* if he couldn't hear the drink a patron ordered in a bar, but there are some pretty rough arguments between editors and writers. Oxford commas, anyone?

When I worked in advertising at a department store a graphic designer casually told me that two spaces didn't belong after a period. We'd worked together for months, and this meant she had to make these small but annoying changes on everything I turned over to her. That she waited so long was a sign of her tact. Now I am obsessed with these two spaces, which originated with the typewriter but have stayed around ever since. Do I judge people who use them? Not exactly, but I notice, like somebody who holds their fork like they're gripping a dagger.

Is it wrong to cast a wary eye at somebody by their punctuation? It matters enough to some people that they send a second text correcting any misspellings in their first text. These are people I might not expect to obsess over such things. Of course some people write to correct your spelling, which is annoying, though your error can easily (too easily!) be blamed on auto-fill.

Technology is supposed to make us clearer, more easily understood, but that is not always the case. We blame spell-check the same way we blame Spotify's algorithm when it plays a song we don't like. (Of course, when Spotify plays a deep track and your friend compliments your taste in music then you accept it with the casual expertise of a person who attended the first CMJ Music Marathon.)

Punctuation is about communication. The same way we notice if somebody is articulate in her speech or in his dress, we notice how they punctuate their emails and texts; a sign of a well-edited mind. Perhaps even more than that. If your punctuation is sloppy, what else in your life is too? Do you keep your dishes in your sink for days on end? Is your bedroom floor littered with dirty clothes? Do you have five thousand emails marked as unread? Is just reading this list making you nervous?

I've had disagreements even with my beloved publisher about commas that finally ended in an uneasy détente. Having strong opinions about commas is something I'm conflicted about. It certainly makes one's life more contentious. Ultimately I enjoy people who speak well and, naturally, write well too. A handwriting test was once common when looking for a job and still happens occasionally in France. You can tell a French person's handwriting at once (the way they write numbers is a giveaway). Or a Japanese person writing English. It's no surprise that those two cultures celebrate process and doing things correctly, which is why they have the best restaurants.

I've always loved the handwriting of anybody I've dated. I think Geoff Dyer wrote in a novel, "love a girl and love her handwriting." Mine, as a left-handed person, is quite difficult. Mostly caps, which is not at all elegant, and I believe a sign, according to people who analyze these things, of a desire for control. That makes sense, I'm afraid. So I've sought pens that are easier for left-handed people to write with. But the aspiration is key. In prose and in public, it's good to care about the mark you leave.

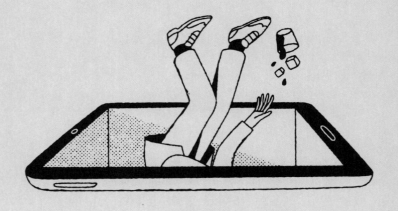

Oversharing

Information Overload

It's amazing how fast the digital realm has evolved. I resisted Facebook for years. Then I realized a lot of artists were sharing information about their shows—these weren't early adapters; they were older painters who discovered a good way to stay connected. I realized, as many do (but perhaps not *quite* enough), that I didn't have to share photos of reunions, pets and meals, and I finally joined. Some friends were surprised. I would have thought you would have a problem with Facebook, they said. Yes, I said with a sigh. It was the worst of both worlds: I was part of something I looked down upon. Then I found out I liked it. Then I found out I didn't need it that much. It was just like anything else; it found its correct level in my life. And that was that.

But a year or so ago, I opened my mom's computer and it was logged into Facebook. "Mom, how long has this been going on?" I asked. This is the woman, after all, who sets her car radio on NPR when she drives it out of the dealership and doesn't change it again. "It was a mistake," she said, "I didn't want to be rude." So now we're all there. Our parents are on Instagram, emoji-fluent, commenting with our friends. Somebody came up to me once and asked if I was David Coggins. Yes, I said, acting like this was normal (it isn't). The man continued, genuinely enthusiastic, "You're David Coggins @drcoggins?" "Um, no . . . that's my father. We have the same name." My dad, who initially resisted Instagram but is now addicted to it, was, of course, thrilled to hear this.

We're still developing codes for how we share our lives. When they go from reality to pixels, some people make their lives fancier. Or sexier. They highlight their nightlife or their dining lives or how much they exercise or, possibly worst of all, their cats. It's all in flux. That's probably why people critique Instagram so much. Some friend always posts champagne, and we complain, wondering, *Do they even drink it?* It's as if we can't decide which bothers us: that our friends were invited to an event that we were not or that they decided to share it.

I like Instagram. I write about travel and am often on the road. I like seeing photos (often taken by strangers) from the Swedish countryside or southwest Texas or people bonefishing on Andros Island. Generally I'm looking for photos I like. I don't really use it to stay close to people, though I understand why people do that. I'd rather connect directly. I want to hear about your life from you, not through a photo.

I like photos of people where they are. Not flashbacks. Not "still dreaming of Paris," though that's personal. There remains a fine line between celebrating a place you're in (or have made a pilgrimage to) and when you treat it like a trophy. "I ate at this sushi temple in Tokyo!" your photo says. It's worth asking if it feels like you're showing off.

These lines are different for different people. But my favorite people on Instagram seem, to a certain extent, to post for themselves. They would be keeping this catalog of photos even in private. In that regard it's a bit like dressing. Of course somebody who's beautifully dressed is communicating something to the public. But the truly brilliant dressers also seem to do it for their own pleasure—as if they would do it in any case. I think that's a guide for Instagram. Don't do it for lifestyle revenge, don't prove you live well (we know you live well!), don't flood the feed and if you see your parent's photo out there, give it a like.

SOCIAL IMPULSES

◆ My feeling about social media is that Instagram and Facebook should be sources of pleasure. Use them in ways that suit you, but also know people will be aware of how you use them. Social media is a way we present ourselves to the world. Like dressing, it's not the most important thing, but it does imply how you see yourself.

◆ Don't get mad if people don't engage with every single thing you do. It's online. It's not real life.

◆ There are endless things I don't like on Instagram: pictures of food, of cats, of watches, of cars. There are sites devoted to just those things and people love them. That's just not for me. I like pictures of travel and architecture, usually without people in them, what my friend calls "boring pictures." Let people have their cult ramen and I'll have Scottish coastlines. There's room for everybody.

◆ However, if you do start sharing your fabulous life people will take your measure by it. So don't misrepresent things. Naturally Instagram can become a fine edit, but try not to brag. The same way you wouldn't in your analog life.

◆ Be aware of how your interaction with your phone and Instagram is affecting those around you. Do you want to delay every meal, every course, with your art-directed overhead shot? Get one shot if you must, then put the phone away and enjoy dinner!

Distraction
In Focus

The older I get the more I appreciate people who are legitimately good at friendship. Not that they're good friends, though they often are, but the actual maintenance of friendship. It's not as easy when you are no longer in school together or banded by age and location. The writer Jim Harrison said that curiosity was the key to friendship—that's what fuels our interest in others. That's what makes us continue to meet people as we get older.

That's certainly true but there's something else: When we are together with our friends, are we actively engaged? Are we listening? Are we taking an interest? Or are we staring at our phones, our minds elsewhere? We've all seen what happens when one person takes their phone out: Everybody else takes a moment to do it as well. And we've all seen tables (or maybe sat at them) that are full of silent, scrolling phone zombies.

My feeling is that the phone peek is something that should happen away from the table. It's as intrusive, in its way, as talking on a phone. We know this is the case, but we feel a vibration or we are expecting an email and then we act on the impulse even when it's against our better judgment. I've adopted a policy that if a friend takes out their phone I just wait in silence until they're finished. This usually communicates that they are interrupting the flow of what we had been sharing.

It's as if we have to learn to make time again. This is another skill. Set up a standing breakfast date you have with a friend, or an annual fishing trip, or have lunch at "21" every few months. I believe in making rituals. If you're lucky, you inherit some, but you'll have to inspire others. So start something. Go to Opening Day, the Village Vanguard, go to the Cloisters. Today can be an occasion. One day you won't remember your life without it.

When we're together, let's make it count. Bring your good material, open that good bottle of wine you've been saving, ask questions and, since you've gone through all that, for goodness' sake, man, pay attention!

GRIEVANCES
This Is Killing Me

PUNCTUATION

"Poor grammar and misused words are my particular peeve. Language is important not for class or educational distinction but because it shows a sense of attention to detail. We taught our sons from an early age to know the difference between 'less' and 'fewer,' or 'if I was' versus 'if I were.' I also think that meaning what you say depends on knowing what you're saying. So when I hear people talking about 'honing in on a problem,' it suggests they aren't thinking about what the words they're using actually mean. *Hone* and *home* are likely the most mixed-up words in business today." —**Chris Mitchell**

DISTRACTION

"The etiquette of cell phones can be frustrating. I don't mean at what times and places it is and isn't appropriate to use them—that should be clear to any reasonable person but apparently isn't. I mean the generational differences in when one calls or texts, for example. When I call a younger person and leave a voice message they'll often reply immediately with a text. And younger people seem to consider it bad manners to call someone without texting them first to ask if it's okay. I suppose technology and communications always change what is and isn't socially acceptable. It used to be appropriate to just go and knock on someone's door unannounced to pay a visit. Now only Jehovah's Witnesses do that." —**Natty Adams**

"Oy, the cell phones! We have to get better with sitting in a group, or one-on-one, or even by ourselves and not heed that siren song of the cell phone. It's so disrespectful at its core. It's saying, 'This little device and whatever is happening on here, is more important than you and [worse!] than my entire surroundings.' It chips away at the beauty of everything—of camaraderie, of conversation, of a museum, of a bar, of a fleeting moment you catch out of the corners of your eyes! And what it has done to dating. These days, we're all just glued to our phones, trying so hard to reach out for a connection by swiping on a godforsaken app. It's like trying to win a football game by throwing the ball through the uprights. It feels like success but it's not getting us anywhere." —**Jacob Gallagher**

"When the conversation comes to a halt because of forgetting names our first inclination is to look it up on our phones. Leave the phone alone, resist the urge to have the knowledge now and keep the conversation going by continuing another side of the subject or using it to ask others what they think. Be creative." —**Christopher DeLorenzo**

SOCIAL MEDIA
Digital Evolution

Chris Black

My friend Chris Black wrote the book *I Know You Think You Know It All* about online behavior, but he was an acknowledged expert long before that. He is legitimately good at Twitter, which turns out to be a rare skill. And he is generally the friend you know will have the right take on all matters social media. I know that if something is important that I need to know about, Chris will let me know. I asked him for his current list of what keeps you in the right, online. —DC

- Don't over-share. We don't need to see or hear it all, just the highlights.

- The selfie is to be avoided. I know it may seem like a good idea and that everyone else is doing it, but stay strong. Something about it reeks of desperation. The likes will not set you free.

- Keep the bragging to a minimum. Sharing your latest work or even the well-intended subtle flex is okay. Outright boasting will leave your audience wanting less.

- Hashtags are a no-no. Hashtags serve a purpose for brands, but they should be left off any posts from your personal accounts. They look amateurish.

◆ Avoid clogging the feed. Got a lot of exciting content? Stay measured and time-release it. Posting five images in a row will annoy even your biggest fans.

◆ Tag someone only when it's flattering. If you are posting a photo from your trip to Lisbon, make sure all parties look good in the chosen image. If someone has clearly overindulged, think twice before sharing. You would want the same courtesy.

◆ Never under any circumstance should you confront someone about unfollowing you. That sort of behavior will make you the talk of the group chat, and not in a good way.

◆ No spoilers. Your uncle in Los Angeles works in the industry and sent you a screener of the latest Oscar-worthy film. Watch it and enjoy it. Do not share any information about said film on social media. Your followers will be mad and so will your uncle.

◆ Be yourself. With so many available platforms to share on, you might slip into a caricature of yourself. Make sure you always keep it real. Don't be someone you aren't—even if you are rewarded with likes and com-ments. Because self-awareness reigns supreme, online and off.

◆ Never take it too seriously. Although social media has become ubiquitous in our modern era, it's still not exactly real life. Hell, maybe put the phone down and take a stroll.

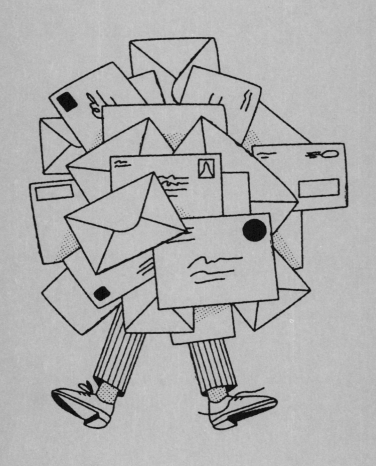

STATIONERY
As Ever

Ted Harrington

Ted has the legacy of being born into the family that operated the longest-running engraved stationery printing press in Manhattan. Now Terrapin Stationers has relocated its HQ to the milder streets of West Haven, Connecticut. But Ted remains a force for propriety and irreverence (a good place to be!). His archives include invitations to film screenings from the 1950s (yes, they engraved those) and more lawyers' pads than you can imagine. Ted loves the Grateful Dead, a healthy amount of swearing, and hates it when *stationery* is misspelled. —DC

It's always a good idea to have a supply of personalized stationery. Engraved, letter-pressed (if you live in Brooklyn) or if you want to save money for drinks, then flat printing is tasteful. If you're not ready for custom, then look for a quality writing paper with matching envelope. Either way, it's time to step away from the MacBook Pro, put down the phone and write a note. By hand. With a pen.

WHERE TO BEGIN
Notecards and envelopes: Go for a white or natural, medium-weight card stock. Nothing too small or too large, (4½" × 6¼" is a good size). Print your first and

last name on the top, and go easy with the nickname. If your name is Charles, then use it. Save Chip for the golf course. Select a classic font, serif or sans serif, and when it comes to ink color, you can't go wrong with blue or black. And don't get carried away with bells and whistles like liners and borders. This set is for business and pleasure. I suggest you skip the return address on the envelope, unless you're going to be writing a lot of notes or staying put for a while.

WHEN TO WRITE

◆ Job interview: Keep it short and professional. Thank you for the interview, it was nice to meet you, I'm interested in learning more, I hope to meet with you again in the near future. With sincere thanks.

◆ Thanks: If someone invites you to their home for the weekend at the shore or for dinner. If you're bringing a bottle for the host, include a note. Thanks for having us. Good for apologies as well. "So sorry about the expletives during dessert . . ."

◆ With sympathy: No one wants to receive a text that reads, "Sorry for your loss."

◆ Just for the hell of it: The best kind of note. I like to go full-on Peter Beard. Cross-outs, write in a circle. Doodles. Blood. Mud. Penis drawing. Whatever.

AT WORK
Clarity and Common Sense

Tony King

Tony is an Englishman in New York. He is an actual creative director in a city full of fake creative directors. His firm, King & Partners, does good work for renowned hotel groups, fashion brands and car companies. It's not surprising that he goes to a lot of meetings (you've probably seen him at a few if you go to breakfast at Lafayette), so I asked him what he thought about office communication. —DC

◆ Use a subject line that lets the recipient know what the email is about—sometimes the subject line can do the job of most of the communication. The email body can be used for details.

◆ Don't use buzzwords.

◆ After finishing the email, go through it and take out any unnecessary words, and replace complicated words with simple words.

◆ Avoid using unnecessary Google docs and spreadsheets; a simple email with a list is far easier for everyone.

◆ Take the time to make sure the email is well written and error-free.

- One thing I always tell my team about meetings: "If you are on time then you are late." Meaning, if the meeting starts at 2pm get there at 1:50pm and be set up to start at 2pm. Don't arrive at 2 and then start at 2:10.

- For new business meetings, 75% of the time should be spent talking about the client, 25% on who you are and what you do. No point spending forty-five minutes out of an hour talking about yourself with no time to ask questions and actually get to discuss the project.

- You can't *not* communicate. Every interaction, every email, everything you send, is communicating something about you, so it has to be thought about, designed, well written, well put together.

"People need to be reminded more often than they need to be instructed."
—Samuel Johnston

THE GUIDELINES

The State of Play for Men Today

Ideas and rules worth remembering. These are not etched in stone. Except for the square-toed shoes—those are never right.

♦   A greeting requires eye contact.

♦   There's no worse way to enter a restaurant than on a phone.

♦   Being good with names is a question of effort, not memory.

♦   As a general rule, people who aren't smoking cigars don't want to be around strangers who are.

♦   Be not the first man to recline his seat.

♦   It's time to buy a second pair of sheets.

♦   You are not going to make any friends by filling the entire overhead bin.

♦   A cigarette butt is litter.

♦   You'll always wish you packed less. Always.

♦   Don't sneeze into your shoulder like a heathen.

♦   Try to avoid asking for the Wi-Fi password for five minutes.

♦   Different people in restaurants have different jobs. Don't hassle the busboy with the waiter's duties.

♦   Buffets are the first step toward anarchy.

- Free champagne is a dangerous thing. Pace yourself.

- Waiters should tell you the price of specials. But there's nothing wrong with asking the market price of something (especially if it involves truffles!). Know what you're getting into so there are no surprises.

- It's not the guide's fault if you're not catching fish.

- Your bag is part of you. If it hits somebody, apologize. (Yet another reason not to wear a backpack in a crowded city.)

- Packing less clarifies your mind and can make you a more expressive dresser.

- When abroad, greet people in their language.

- Tip well but remember what author Gérard Oberlé said: "Friendship cannot be purchased with a tip."

- People notice when you check your phone.

- Not everybody has the same email and text habits you do. If it's not business related, give them time.

- Let he who texts not cast the first unsolicited photo.

- You're old enough to give money to a charity or arts organization. Even if it's only $25.

- No matter your level of expertise, don't order wine without consulting the rest of the table. Unless you're hosting and settling the tab.

- Every handwritten note is appreciated.

- "We all had a lot to drink" is usually said by the drunkest person in the room. And is not a good excuse for bad behavior.

- Nobody wins in the comments section.

- An exclamation point in a text can be your ally.

- You don't want to finish your meal before your date finishes hers. Overzealous staff might clear your dish and then you're left staring at her.

- Nobody ever won an argument in a sports bar.

- A napkin is not a handkerchief.

- It's good to have an unpredictable interest.

- If you can't drive a stick shift you'll regret it at the most inopportune time.

- If you're useful in the kitchen it will pay off regularly.

- Don't fear subtitles.

- If you must wear a baseball hat, wear your home team and never backward.

- When you can afford to hire a housekeeper then try it.

- Women will judge your sheets, towels and furniture. And rightly so.

- Nobody is your bro.

- No reason to lie to your tailor, fishing guide, doctor, caddy or your mother. They'll find out the truth soon enough.

- If there's a line outside think twice.

- You already know you should look at your phone less.

- There's nothing wrong with asking for advice in a good men's store, even if you can't afford to shop there. They'll be more helpful than you realize.

- Ask your grandparents what life was like fifty years ago and don't interrupt them.

- You have to start cooking sometime. Mark Bittman's recipes from his Minimalist column are a great place to start. (They're all on the *New York Times* website.)

- You'll never regret being a regular.

- Beware white or black socks in public, unless you're playing tennis or attending a funeral.

- You're not ready for a night out without any cash.

- Have a calling card made that you're proud of, your name and number are enough.

- Donate to your favorite museum in your city.

- Fantasy football misaligns your allegiances.

- Two posts a day on Instagram are probably enough.

- Don't exalt Patrick Bateman, even ironically.

- If something will fit when you lose weight then it doesn't fit.

- A logo impresses nobody you want it to impress.

- Rent and salary are private matters.

- Your dry cleaner can hem your pants, but anything more than that requires a tailor. Find one you trust; they'll solve countless problems. Ignacio's on E. 60th Street in Manhattan is a good start.

- Use "work emergency" as an excuse sparingly.

- Your friend referred a client to you? Send them a good bottle of scotch.

- In a crowded bar don't save a seat for somebody who hasn't arrived.

- When talking to sommeliers, be specific about your tastes and tell them how much to spend. Nothing to be ashamed of if you're looking for a good value—good sommeliers are proud of their rare or obscure bottles, and happy to share them with you.

- People want to hear about your vacation—up to a point. A highlight and a lowlight will do.

- If you can't make a dinner reservation, call and tell them. Even if it's only half an hour before.

- Do everything in your power not to rent clothes.

5

Dating

Going Out

The Dating Game

May you live in interesting times. Is this true for dating as well? There are countless choices when you're trying to meet the one. We can swipe left, find fellow fetishists and meet people who are in the mood. You can take the analog approach and buy somebody a drink. There are many options but not a lot of protocol. If you clear the basic hurdle then you might be lucky enough to date a woman who is more successful than you are. Congratulations!

But then do you pay the bill? There are conflicting messages. We want to be sympathetic, enlightened men who are deeply familiar with the menu at Sqirl. But it's nice to hold a door open, to treat a meal, to show some chivalry.

I don't pretend to have the answer. In general I pay for the first meal no matter who I'm with. I think it sets a tone whether you're with a woman you're attracted to or a man who you want to be friends with. I also think a woman deserves the better seat and a certain amount of deference. But my God, let her choose the wine if she's so inclined. If she wants to pay the bill don't fight over it. I always find it attractive when a woman pays. Though I treat her next time. And hopefully there is a next time.

A certain clear-headedness is welcome. Try to imitate a man you admire, and things will fall in line. It's the same when it comes to dressing. Do you want to be the most underdressed man in the room? Of course not. You want to dress in a way where you won't be embarrassed if you see a photo years later.

I have to say I'm too old to have been in the trenches with online dating. It doesn't appeal to my slow-moving tastes. Which is not to say I haven't looked over a friend's shoulder as he was swiping this way and that or chose the background music to his profile. It was fascinating! Like watching Mexican wrestling—it was a spectacle that nobody seemed to take too seriously, and everybody was wearing a mask, so to speak. I've also ghost-written a few texts to my friends' love interests, while they've looked on. It was liberating!

Conversation and words appeal to me. So does a strong will and a pretty face. Under very different circumstances Abigail Adams told her son, John Quincy, above all, "Don't be a blockhead." What was true for the future president is true for us now. Hold the door, defer, look her in the eye. But missteps happen. Of course they do—uncertainty and attraction are involved.

Yes, the history of dating is littered with embarrassments. For those of us who grew up watching *Fast Times*, it was Rat forgetting his wallet while they had one soda after another in that scary German restaurant in the mall. These things happen at any age. But try to do the right thing, and more often than not, you'll come out the other side with everybody's dignity intact.

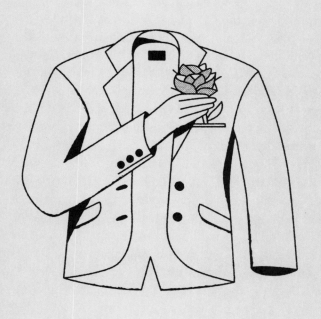

First Dates

Dating could be a whole book and not one I would like to write. But here are some things that I've learned in twenty years of living in New York. Some lessons arrived the easy way, the hard way or the embarrassing *I hope I never see this person as long as I live* way.

I think in general it's better to be direct. If you like somebody, ask them out. Not to vaguely hang out sometime, but specifically on a date for a drink or for dinner. If you go to a bar please don't go anywhere that has a television. You're there to talk and get closer, not to watch a baseball game over her shoulder. Also, the place should serve wine that's not embarrassing to order. Plenty of women prefer a glass of red or white to beer or spirits.

By now I hope you know this bar. But if not, it shouldn't be so loud you can't converse. And hopefully it's near a restaurant that you like in case you want to go there afterward (it could even be in a restaurant itself, if you just want to stay at the bar and eat). It doesn't have to be a major production, you don't need molecular gastronomy. Freemans in New York is good. I like sitting at restaurant bars on a date, it feels less intense. Then pay the bill. Doesn't mean you're behind the times, doesn't mean she owes you anything, just settle the tab, say it was your pleasure.

Today you can learn a lot about a woman before you meet her in person. Google, Instagram and the rest of it. You can see if somebody has mutual friends, was an extra in a sitcom or ever had a punk phase. This is tricky because when you finally meet, you have to decide to divulge just how much research you did ahead of time. In a sense, you want to strike the right balance—what man wouldn't want to show enough interest to know that his date wrote a great piece in *Vanity Fair*? But you don't want to have gone onto her sister's Instagram feed to find out what her childhood home looks like.

Sometimes these situations arrive before you can plan them. I was out with a woman, and I couldn't help learning from the Internet (which is to say I looked her up on Google) that she had been married to a man in a popular band. When she casually said that she was divorced, I tried to bluff my way through by saying very slowly, "Oh really?" I should have just said, "Right, I saw that. I was curious about you and looked it up." Since she could certainly tell anyway. But I do think people deserve a certain amount of time to reveal their life to you. Don't bring up a divorce or their child or anything else before they do. How we reveal information about ourselves is a form of intimacy.

Not every date ends in a kiss. I'm sure you know this. But I certainly have suffered the dreaded unintentional kiss, when a woman leans in clearly (in retrospect) with the intention of kissing me politely on the cheek, only to find my mouth there. This is not ideal. It's far less than ideal, in fact. Though there are embarrassments that can be even worse. But it happens. And hopefully things go better the next time.

I am for texting the next day. I don't care about what they said in *Swingers* about waiting three days to call. If you like her, tell her. Get to the phase of straight talk as soon as possible. By straight talk I don't mean you're announcing your political beliefs—there's time for mystery—just that there's no reason to try to be clever and act like you don't care. In any case caring is good because it can lead to much better things. And that's the point, isn't it?

Breaking Up

End of the Affair

Most of the best things in life happen in the physical world and away from screens: Lunch at Le Grand Véfour, landing a large brown trout, seeing the Giotto frescoes in Santa Croce. Of course, the bad ones happen in person too. That's the nature of things. When it's time to end a relationship, it has to be done with eye contact. Not over the phone, not in an email and certainly not by fleeing the scene altogether ("ghosting," in the parlance of our times).

What makes it difficult is, naturally, what makes it necessary. If you're afraid of tears or a scene, choose your location carefully, but choose one in the real world. I'm not going to tell you how to break up, other than be short and direct (but not so direct you list any shortcomings). It's not a time to revisit old arguments, though gravity will pull you toward that, so beware.

There's no formula any more than there's a formula for how to be broken up with. When I took it on the romantic chin once I just lay down on the couch and listened to Low's early records on repeat (Duluth's finest band plays sad, unhurried songs that are tailor-made for the slow burn). Actually, it was before I had a couch, it was more of a loveseat (oh cruel name!), and so I couldn't stretch all the way out, just curl up in the fetal position.

(On the subject of being broken up with, once this happened to me in the London townhouse of my girlfriend at the time. She lived on the top floor, and I had to leave in ignominy in the morning, my trip having been cut short as it were. As I tried to leave under cover of stealth I ran into her mother as I was walking out the front door. She looked me up and down, noted my luggage and rather wistfully asked if I was checking out.)

These things happen to us, and hopefully we don't have to inflict them on others, but when called upon do it right. Don't minimize the situation (none of this "we were never official, anyway")—you know when the end is nigh, and the sooner you clarify and finalize things the better for all involved. Sometimes the bell tolls for thee; have the decency to do the difficult thing face-to-face.

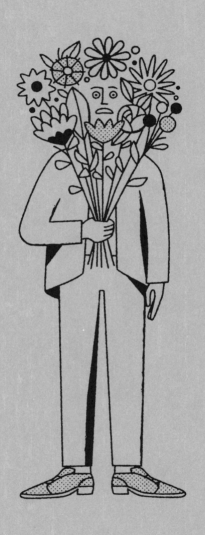

DATING BY THE NUMBERS
No Excuses

Jon Birger

Jon Birger is the journalist who wrote *Date-onomics: How Dating Became a Lopsided Numbers Game*. I wanted more than anecdotal evidence, so here are the numbers that explain his theories about what's wrong with men on the town these days. —DC

Date-onomics explains why dating nowadays is so much harder for women than for men—particularly for college-educated women. In other words: Why is it that so many women in their thirties and forties have *everything* going for them dating-wise yet struggle with dating, even as mildly appealing men never seem to stay single for more than five minutes?

Well, my argument is that this is not a strategic problem but a demographic one. For the past fifteen years in the United States (and in most Western countries), we've had four women graduate from college for every three men. The end result is a post-college dating pool with 33% more college-grad women than college-grad men. *That* is the man deficit in a nutshell. According to Census data, there are about 5.5 million college-grad women in the United States who are age 22–29 versus only 4 million men. Of course, this wouldn't matter so much if we were all more open-minded about whom we date and eventually marry. But the research on this shows that we aren't open-minded at all. There's been a long-term trend in the United States toward what sociologists call "assortative mating"—which is a fancy way of saying that college grads tend to want only to date and marry other college grads. For men, this bias against working-class (or non-college-grad) women does not cost them because the supply of college-grad women is so vast. But for college-grad women, the unwillingness to date non-college-grad men has a high cost. Not only are those women limiting themselves to a too-small dating pool, but it allows college-grad men to act badly. Those guys know they're in high demand, and a lot of them act accordingly. Indeed, the key argument of *Date-Onomics* is that the rise of the hookup culture and the declining marriage rates of college-grad women are both by-products of lopsided sex ratios among the college educated.

The reason men—particularly college-grad men— behave badly is because the market conditions promote it. In fact, there's been a lot of scholarly research on how sex ratios impact human behavior, and the consensus is that the dating culture is looser and less monogamous when women are in oversupply. Men are more likely to have multiple sex partners and less likely to remain committed to the same partner throughout her child-bearing years.

ONLINE ROMANCE
Some Analysis

Ty Tashiro

Ty Tashiro is the only person in this book (as far as I know) who has a PhD, which gives him the authority to discuss a vitally important topic: how technology has affected social interaction and dating. He's the author of *Awkward: The Science of Why We're Socially Awkward and Why That's Awesome*. He discusses his research about the new landscape of dating. I was interested in his thoughts on texting and meeting, the digital and the analog, and getting to know somebody in real time. —DC

ONLINE DATING

Colleagues of mine who work as researchers at some of the biggest online dating sites all say the same thing about the objective of online dating: "The app is a means to an end, and that end is getting face-to-face with someone." A well-behaving gentleman does not languish in texting territory for weeks on end; rather, he sees texting as a way to exchange some niceties, then arrange for a face-to-face meeting that allows both parties to comfortably interact at a reasonable hour of the evening.

One of the biggest effects of online dating on human mating behavior has been the explosion of perceived possibility. A quick behavioral economics lesson puts this in perspective. When economists try to predict when people will buy or sell a stock, house or other asset, they look at three factors: What kind of value does the person expect, how well does their current investment do, and how do they perceive the value of alternative investments available?

These same three factors do a great job of predicting when people will commit or break up with a romantic partner. What has happened in the online dating era is that singles' awareness of the available alternative dating options has skyrocketed, which has kind of broken the dating algorithm in people's minds.

The result has been widespread bad behavior, especially on the part of men who feel free to ghost, breadcrumb or engage in a number of other behaviors that suggest they do not see dates in people of value. It may be true that the number of dating options has exponentially increased in recent years thanks to online dating, and that a few swipes can generate a great deal of possibility, but this convenience does not excuse bad behavior, which inevitably has an impact on a real person with real feelings.

ONGOING RELATIONSHIPS

Once there is an "us" between two people, technology provides numerous opportunities for downright crazy behavior. In the context of human relationships, romantic relationships represent the highest level of difficulty and the highest emotional stakes. Whenever there are high psychological stakes, people become extremely attentive to the smallest signals that something might be amiss, which is why partners are so easily driven mad by a delayed response to a text or a partner's photo on Instagram with a suspiciously beautiful stranger.

You can use technology to drive your partner crazy, but it inevitably starts a cycle of bad behavior in which everyone loses. We need to use technology in a timely and responsive manner because we know that there are outsized effects from the uncertainty created by being unresponsive or cryptic. For those of us prone to anxiety or obsessiveness, it's also important to take a few deep breaths when we're reading too far into hiccups in communication that does not happen face-to-face.

After all, it's unnatural for people in intimate relationships to communicate through devices. The human mind has evolved over thousands of years to make use of nonverbal behaviors, scent, tone of voice, touch and a host of other cues that are removed when people communicate through their phones.

Once again, technology is a means, not an end, when it comes to matters of the heart.

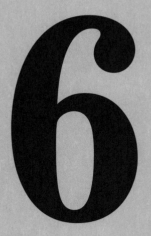

Travel

THE GAUNTLET
PLANES
HOTELS
VISITING
RIGHT-THINKING PEOPLE

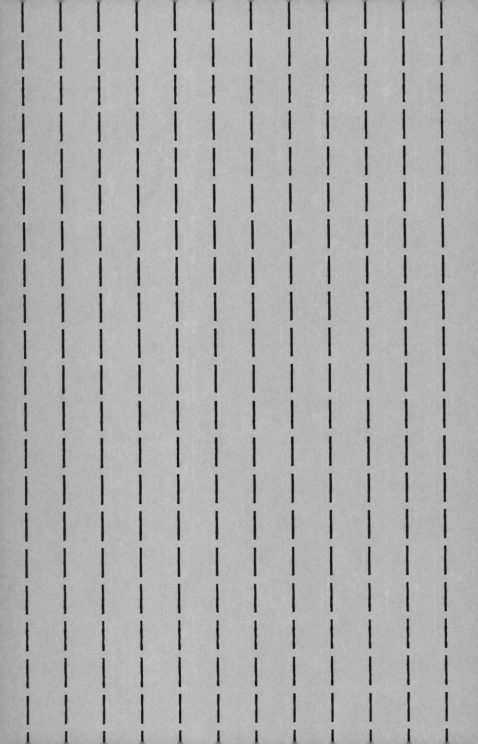

The Gauntlet

Survival Tactics

Travel is the gauntlet, the supreme test. Can you keep it together through security and boarding and overhead bins and maintain your dignity and your temper? Somehow it's devolved into a free-for-all, belts and shoes are coming off, people are trying to wheel on bags the size of shopping carts, and then when you finally settle in, somebody asks to switch seats with you. We can blame greedy airlines and their endless fees, we can blame the security follies, but we also have to blame human nature.

No doubt you've developed tactics for the trenches. But here's a call not to race to the bottom. Men traveling for business seem to conduct that business everywhere and at full volume. Airport lounges seem to attract men who feel comfortable participating in a phone meeting at full blast. Please do not be one of those men.

More than anywhere else, when you're traveling, a little kindness goes a long way. Probably because people are wearing tracksuits and getting into arguments with strangers while lying on the ground. It's not that hard: Travel in a sportcoat, with not too much baggage, and smile. This formulation is easy to master and will endear you to flight attendants, gate check staff and your fellow travelers. A recent article in the *Times* said that certain airlines allow their gate check staff to upgrade polite, well-dressed people. That chance alone should be all the encouragement you need. But allow me to offer some more.

If you are not spending all your time worrying about the overhead bins your life will be a lot better. If you are going to descend into the fray then at least keep in mind that most issues will be resolved sooner rather than later. We've all lost luggage and have our horror stories, not every travel situation is a zero-sum, pitched battle.

Yes, there are jerks who take up the entire overhead bin with two bags and their jackets (evil!). But don't try to enforce everything. Travel light. From a dressing point of view, you'll be surprised how little you need when you're abroad. A clean edit, with a few accessories, really helps develop your sense of dressing. Fabric with a little heft to it (as opposed to really fine cotton and wool) is good. Oxford shirts are ideal since they don't wrinkle much and dry easily. Washing a shirt in your hotel room is within your skills as a gentleman.

When you travel, you see people who seem to have made the airport their home. They spread out on the concourse like they're having a picnic. They seem to have found food you didn't know existed. Couples abandon their children to bright drinks and loud games on their computers.

This is not you. You are the man with a wry expression and a kind word for everybody he deals with. You communicate to all that you understand the absurdity of modern travel and rise above it. You have a sense of decorum but don't enforce every rule when some heathen tries to board ahead of his zone number. When you travel, the most important thing to bring is a good sportcoat and a sense of proportion.

TRAVEL ETIQUETTE
Local Knowledge

♦ Under no circumstances should you bring hot food into an airplane or a train car. (They should really frog-march anybody who does this right off the plane and out of polite society.)

♦ Wait until they call your zone. Some people act uncertain about which zone was called and merge with the first-class travelers. You know who you are.

♦ Don't bombard your seat neighbor with conversation. "So where's home?" "What line of work are you in?" When you hear these warning signs, you may be sitting next to somebody—usually, but not exclusively, a man in sales—keen to chat. A smile, a polite answer and then a return to your book. Follow up with a question at your own risk.

♦ Very specific to those in New York: Do not sit on the busy steps of Grand Central. You couldn't be more in the way. This is true of other landmarks and travel hubs. Just because someplace looks inviting does not mean you should spread yourself upon it.

♦ Reverse advice: The most predictable advice is that you shouldn't drink on a plane. It, as we all know, dehydrates you. This is crazy: Drinking on a plane (particularly on a long flight) is perfectly enjoyable. Don't pound a Bloody Mary on a 7am flight, but a drink on an overseas flight is most welcome.

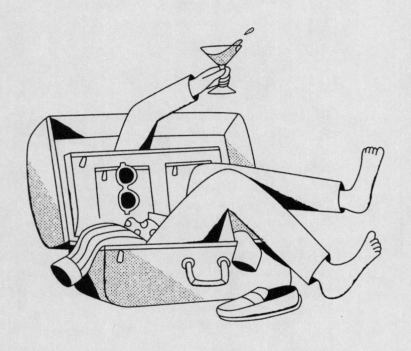

Planes
Laid Low

Are there unknown strategies left to make flying better? You can have status on an airline. You can pack light—and I mean light. You can game it around the edges and get lucky. Save money or time or make it into a lounge. But I think the best thing you can do is just exhale. Things won't always be ideal, but expect that in advance. In many cases you're talking about a few extra minutes in line. Of course there are fiascos on runways and four-hour waits and then they run out of food.

But in general, see it as a test of your patience, resolve and good cheer. One problem with flying is the thinly veiled anarchy that encourages a free-for-all: Do what you have to do to charge your phone at the gate, then "merge" into the line whether or not your zone has been called—whatever it takes to get your bag in the overhead. And while you're doing all this, some business traveler is having a conversation at full volume as if they're completely alone in a conference room. Meanwhile somebody else is trying to put a roller bag the size of a phone booth into the overhead bin.

You get these people telling you to drink plenty of water—is there a more common bit of advice anywhere? Don't drink on planes, they say. Don't drink? I fly Air France because they serve Armagnac after meals. And I have to tell you, I've done a lot of writing after those Armagnacs—enough to make it my bureau in the sky.

Flying will never be perfect. You can't reeducate everybody. You can just try to have a small footprint. Small bag overhead, a second one underneath, smile to the flight attendant. Be the bright spot. Don't put your seat back if you're sitting in the front row. And don't monopolize the armrests. Those belong to the sad people in the center seats.

You are the cheerful warrior. And the fact that the world does not reach the heights of your ideal standard does not excuse descending into the scrum as you reach cruising altitude.

Hotels
Checking In

I remember how liberating it was to read Guy Trebay write in the *Times* a while back that he was a serial hotel room redecorator. When he checked in on one of the stops on his European fashion week circuit, he would deposit unwanted artwork in the closet, rearrange furniture. In short, he made the place his own. Inspired!

I do think it's good to really move in. Hide the ridiculous magazines. Have them remove the contents of the minibar if you're not a drinker (not at all uncommon in the Chateau Marmont, I gather). Then get to know the concierge. In a foreign city they are a valuable weapon in your arsenal. Give them a clear idea of what type of bar or restaurant or cultural outing you're looking for; like talking to a tailor or sommelier, it's good to be specific. And let them know how it was. Even if it wasn't the best, they want to be informed. In Tokyo, I've talked to concierges three times a day about traditional sushi restaurants, Kyoto temples, ceramic stores, newly appealing neighborhoods. I write them before I arrive and we plot—this is a ground operation! I realize I'm on the obsessive end of things, but endearing yourself to the staff can only be a good thing.

What's true of restaurants is also true of hotels, the more people you know by name, the better. If you get into the spirit of a place and are warm toward the people who work there, then they will remember and respond to you. When you get to the personal side of a business, then you are on the right side of it. I've had a habit of frequenting cafés and bars and restaurants since I was studying abroad and was old enough to choose them for myself. I recommend this practice in the strongest possible terms.

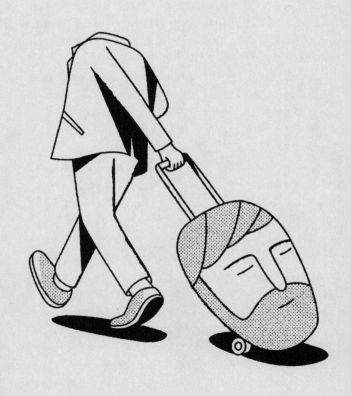

Does it mean leaving money for the concierge? It does. Does it mean writing a letter to the hotel after you've left? It can. When you are familiar enough with the manager that you email him for a room the next time you're going to visit, then you are in the right position.

Even if you rearrange things, remember: You're not a rock star; don't trash anything. Leave no mess behind, just a tip for the maid.

Visiting
Make
Yourself
at Home

When you're twenty and you visit a friend in college, all you get is a couch, and you repay the favor with a few pitchers of bad beer. When you're older, you get a bed (unless you live in New York, in which case it's still the couch), and the stakes are raised.

Perhaps you take your friend to dinner. Maybe a bottle of scotch upon arrival. But you're not in college anymore. No matter your age, you want to leave as small a footprint as possible. You like to scatter your clothes around your own bedroom? That's fine, but you're not in your bedroom. In fact, your habits are now secondary to your host's.

Of course, a good host does his best to make you feel comfortable. But when somebody says, "Make yourself at home," they mean it only up to a point. You don't want to put up any speed bumps to their routine. You don't convert the dining room table into your mobile office. You don't impose your early-morning playlists on unsuspecting late risers.

A meal is the best thing you can offer. Eggs on Sunday morning are usually welcome. A simple supper, if that makes sense. Bring some nice food and then prepare it. You want your host to benefit the way you're benefiting. A simple rule is usually effective: Arrive with a gift. Send a note (or an email, if that's your game) the next day by noon. If a household needs something (tools for the Weber, a big cutting board, a nice wine opener), then send one on. A useful present is welcome, especially if it's just a little nicer than it needs to be (which is why there are German knives and Japanese teapots).

If you're a houseguest for a weekend then we're talking even more. Propose to cook a meal ahead of time. Consult your host about what's in the kitchen and bring whatever else

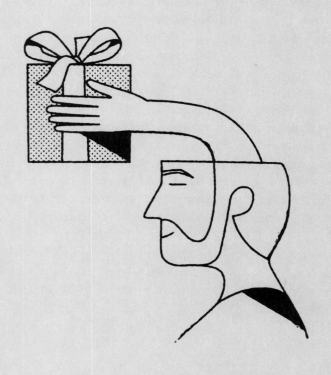

you need, and bring enough to drink for the weekend. Err on the side of an extra bottle. Get involved in dishwashing. It's an easy way to get in the spirit. If, however, the host likes having the kitchen to himself or herself then take a hint and give some space. Not every chef likes a full kitchen.

Get in the spirit of how the house operates. If your hosts don't follow sports then don't watch an MLB doubleheader. If your team is in the playoffs and you're the type of fan who paints his face (which I doubt) then perhaps you need to reconsider your priorities. You're not there to follow along on your device; you're there to spend time with your friends away from the distractions of technology.

A good host replies in kind. They tell you where the coffee is and how to make it. They let you choose a record. And, of course, you return the offer. If you stay in somebody's house while they're away then there should be something nice waiting for them upon their return. Not to be coldhearted about it, but those warm feelings are what get you invited back. On a more basic level, it's the debt we pay to friendship.

GRIEVANCES
This Is Killing Me

"It drives me crazy when an impatient passenger onboard a crowded plane, which has landed but before the door has opened, insists on pushing forward past others. It's both pointless and rude." —**Dewey Nicks**

"Carrying a full-size bed pillow onto a commercial aircraft." —**Chris Benz**

"If you have a airline credit card, you probably have a free checked bag—use that perk. Doesn't cost you anything, and it makes traveling infinitely easier. Travel is stressful enough." —**Nick Roberts**

"My biggest issue with traveling is the lack of patience and tolerance most people have for one and other. I would love to see more people ask an elderly women to place her luggage in the overhead compartment, or hold the door for someone rather than looking at their phone. Awareness has gone by the wayside." —**Javas Lehn**

"In security it shouldn't be a surprise that you have to take off your shoes, so wear shoes that easily slip on and off." —**Kirk Miller**

"Airport restaurants that only let you order on an iPad are the Epcot Center of dining."—**Matt Stiles**

RIGHT-THINKING PEOPLE

A Conversation with Mark Rozzo

Do you have a friend who does a lot of things suspiciously well? So well that if you didn't really like him, you wouldn't be able to stand him? Yes? Then perhaps you know Mark as well, because it seems that everybody knows him. He is a writer, editor, teacher, and he's in a band (that's actually good). He is also a devoted father, well-dressed, and, I'm sorry to report, handsome as well. Basically he's the worst. And of course the best—which is why I wanted to hear his thoughts on men and matters and society today. —DC

What did you learn from your father? What rules did he have?
My dad was a man of few words. But he was a big man, with a big man's quiet dignity. He never sat me down and said, "Son, these are the rules of the road" in some cheeseball way. He led by example. If you're mowing the lawn, make sure you get the job right when you're working around the trees. When you sink a basket, don't gloat or showboat. The guy rarely lost his cool, despite the pressures of an often high-pressure career. In some ways, I'm more like my hot-under-the-collar, slightly harried mother, but the reserve, the respect, the patience, the attention to detail, the basic decency: That was him in a nutshell (maybe his generation in a

nutshell), and a lot of rules follow from that outlook.
I do my best with it, but I'll never nail it like he did.

**What do you think about manners today? Do you have a
particular pet peeve?**

Pet peeves are my main pet peeve, so I try not to be
driven crazy by everybody else's limitless shortcomings.
The stuff that bothers me bothers all right-thinking
people: leaving a crappy tip, trying to jump the green
light at an intersection, really anything that smacks of
impatience and a lack of generosity or cooperation. And
using *I* as a direct object ("She gave her suntan lotion to
Charlie and I."), which I know is more about linguistic
usage than politeness, but there's a moral dimension to
treating the language like shit. And then there's lateness, which is a whole category until itself. I'm afraid to
say that I've lost probably entire months of my life waiting around for a friend, one who's been as close to me as
any other human for the past thirty-plus years. Not sure
what kind of demerit I get for continuing to be friends
with this person or not exploding in rage often enough,
but that kind of response feels somehow . . . impolite.

Facebook inherently offends me. The branding of
the self, the corporatization of the soul, the free play
in the scrum of ego and envy, the pimping of cute
offspring in order to gain "likes." I find it breaks every
known dictum of acceptable, tasteful behavior. So I
don't participate. I'm also probably too insecure and
afraid of judgment to have an account.

Another thing I find rude and tasteless is when
artists, authors, chefs and the like "talk back" to their

critics; have some pity on the poor critic, forced to sift through the culture week to week, trying to find something wonderful to extol.

Do you have any questions about etiquette or manners that you keep coming back to?
Have you noticed that in the UK and Ireland people on the street attempt to pass you on your right? In the United States, we always pass on the left, the way we do on the highway. This causes endless sidewalk confusion! I'm pretty sure I'm not dreaming this up. Can someone clarify that the origins of this phenomenon are rooted in the respective road habits of these countries?

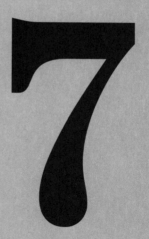

Conflict

APOLOGIES
FRICTION
ARGUING
PEEVES

Apologies
Take Your Medicine

Sometimes you have to say I'm sorry. It should be simple but rarely is. Somebody else started it. Everybody was drunk. It was taken out of context. Whatever. The situation was nuanced. But the apology shouldn't be. Just make it direct.

I've had to apologize for many things. Some were foolish on my part. Other times I thought people were too sensitive. But if you make your sister cry on her birthday, which I'm ashamed to say I've done, then it doesn't matter if you were *technically* right. There is no right when you make somebody cry, even if the table is littered with empty wine bottles. I've apologized in person, by text, by email, in apartments, in corporate offices. I'd like to think that I've gotten good at it, but if you are good at apologizing then you are offending too many people. In the end, you have to keep it to the point—it's important to say the words. It acknowledges your mistake, your contrition. Then you move on.

None of this "I'm sorry if I offended you"—at that point you clearly did offend the person. If the thing that's standing between you and a friendship is an apology, that is not a major thing. You can even apologize in a fight and not be entirely at fault. It's not a zero-sum circumstance. Your counterpart might apologize as well. It can be therapeutic, but the stubbornness (I've had it myself) is an important thing to overcome.

Sometimes a quick word about something that seems minor is the best solution. If you realize you have called somebody the wrong name, say, "George, I'm sorry I called you Jeff earlier." Be assured that every time somebody is called an incorrect name, they remember it. They are also quick to forgive.

Wrong names are not the end of the world, but I've made far more major errors that were quite public. When I was working in the advertising department for a celebrated department store in New York, every day we sent out an email to our mailing list. That's hundreds of thousands of people. Somehow in the subject line I typed the designer Derek Lam's name as "Derek Lamb." Naturally spell-check didn't save me, since "lamb" is a word (another example of trusting technology to save us from ourselves). This was not good. The president was involved. The corporate office. They changed protocols. It's true that there were people who should have caught this, but the entire thing started with me.

It quickly became clear it was my fault. And the round of apologies was thorough. I was reminded about showing contrition and being direct. Will it surprise you that all the higher-ups were very forgiving? They were certainly not happy, but they all understood that people make honest mistakes and they saw I was sorry. It's also a reminder that there's an art to accepting an apology. Forgiveness, like apologies, can be short and to the point.

There are thoughts about what's the best way to apologize. Sometimes it has to be done in writing. The situation is just too hot. Or it's a professional matter and a number of executives are cc'd. Sometimes it has to be done face-to-face (difficult, of course!). But don't explain so much that your central message is watered down. *I'm sorry I did this. This is what I was thinking, which I realize was wrong. I shouldn't have done it.* Of course in the moment, everything heats up, you have to face the person and say it directly.

If you disappeared from a woman's life—what the kids call "ghosting"—then a simple apology is not going to be enough. She will rightly want to know that you learned something and that you've changed. Before heading down the path of apology you should ask yourself if those things are true and if you are you ready to do the right thing beyond saying sorry. People can always tell if your sorry isn't that sorry at all—or as Kramer memorably said to a reluctantly apologetic George: "I'm sorry, I don't care for that sorry."

Some people are under the impression that you never concede an error, that it shows weakness or some other unflattering quality. I don't see that at all. It shows you're human and, if anything, it makes you a more evolved person. A relationship that doesn't involve forgiveness is not very intimate to begin with.

Friction

Know Your Audience

On the first day of a fishing trip my guide asked me about my opinion of a particular seismic political event. Feeling we were sympathetic I replied that it was awful. This came as a surprise to him, and the fact that he celebrated this event (which had caused me such anguish) was just as much a surprise to me. In fact, I was fishing to avoid thinking about the flaws of civilization, not revisit them.

But once the topic was brought up I should have hedged. How do I know what the guide thinks of politics? It's a classic case of assuming sympathetic people agree with you. Better to give a measured response and move on. There's a time to dig into the political trenches (and a way to do it), and there's a time to avoid it.

This is true of all sorts of cultural friction. I'm often in the minority when it comes to some cultural phenomenon, which is why I would never wait in line to buy some streetwear collaboration. Delivering a withering opinion is an art that's rarely practiced well. You loathed the Whitney Biennial? You think *Game of Thrones* is overrated? You have any thought at all on *Girls*? Hey now, people are paying attention. But in most cases the gentle knife is more effective than the hatchet.

Nobody wants to be on the receiving end of a diatribe, whether it's against the evils of a political party or the star of a rival team. As I get older, I admire more and more the subtlety of somebody who can disagree with discretion. One clever tactic is to repeat your opinion back to you with a lingering question: "Oh, you liked the *Twin Peaks* return?" There's no attack. They give you space. You can pursue the discussion if you like, temper your remark, or just move on.

One unfortunate situation about the current state of affairs is that we become so dismissive of people on the other side of the political aisle that we state our moral objections up front. Some things don't need to be discussed straightaway. In fact, generally it's better to avoid politics with strangers. Too often we just want to recite our thoughts as if the matter will end there. Well of course it doesn't end there. Not everything has to be solved in every conversation. You are not less of a believer if you don't trot out your favorite lines about the tax code or whatever else it is. We need more diplomats on a daily basis, more people who have convictions but don't need to fight it out until it really matters. Not everything is at stake at every moment in the day, even though it often feels like it.

Sometimes it's a situation when you stand up for something; sometimes you fight another day. But remember that in a complicated world there's always room for error. Some of those errors might be yours.

Arguing
Debate
Society

It's hard to win an argument. In fact, I'm starting to think nobody has ever won one. By the time you're angry and raising your voice, it's too late to change anybody's mind—they've dug in and are just set on rebutting you. LeBron vs. Michael, *Sopranos* vs. *Mad Men*, hearing yourself say, "We never said we were exclusive." Your mind, of course, doesn't need changing—you have the burden of being serially correct (Michael, *Sopranos*, you never said this). Regardless of who's right then, there are better ways of persuasion than friction.

I'm definitely not perfect in the debate department. I even enjoy a little vigorous debate from time to time, and when I was younger, quite a lot. But when I look back at bad moments in my life they are almost always arguments that got out of control. More than that, once they escalate, they always seem to be more about some larger disagreement than the issue at hand.

This is something to remember in our private lives—nearly everybody is more open to suggestions when they are proposed calmly. But it's also true in public—when you are artfully registering your dissatisfaction with the maître d' don't put him on the back foot.

I aspire to a life without arguments. I'm not sure that's possible. In fact, I am certain it is not. But I think we can be more persuasive without them. More than that, I think we can be happier and better versions of ourselves when we're not trying to prove that we're right, not trying to convince somebody else the error of their ways. When you take the long view, there's a chance for common ground, less resistance and a better way all around.

Peeves
Cover Thy Feet

Tolerance is good. Giving people the benefit of the doubt: also good. Pacing up and down an otherwise quiet airport lounge conducting a meeting as if it's your private office, as if you're not surrounded by countless other business travelers? Less forgivable. But, for me, if there's something that borders on the etched-in-stone inexcusable, it has to do with feet.

There is no tradition of a man's feet in art. No Renaissance marble slab commissioned by the Medici of hairy toes. They're not an object of beauty. All of which is to say: Don't wear flip-flops in public. Not even your loved ones find your toes attractive. Choose your footwear accordingly.

If you're on the beach, of course, do what needs doing. But for heaven's sake, when you're in town, when you're at restaurants, when you're on *a plane*, keep your feet covered. It's remarkable the bubble people enter into that makes them feel like they're in private when they're not. Just because you wear noise-canceling headphones does not mean you are in your living room.

The line between public and private is one of the foundations of society. Pride yourself on your honesty, that's fine, but that doesn't mean you should speak on your cell phone loudly enough that everybody else knows what you think you'll have for dinner.

If you're in Japan then this goes without saying. They have their sanitary priorities in order and keep bare feet covered in socks. I'm not sure about this impulse to need to be relaxed and comfortable at all times. This happens to children who don't want to take off their superhero pajamas when they have to go to school. But we're not boys anymore.

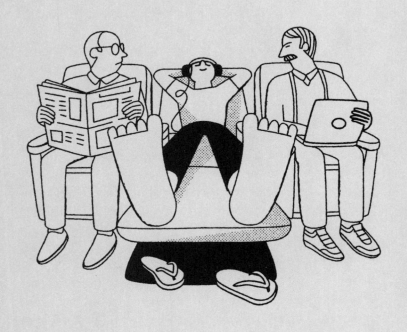

There are more elevated ways to be comfortable than wearing a tracksuit. In fact, one of your challenges is to be at your ease without looking like you're not fit for society.

Even for those of us who go sockless, I slip on socks before wandering up the aisles of a plane. Your feet are nobody's business but your own.

MORE PEEVES
A Few Things off My Chest

So much of this book is about not getting bogged down in the excruciating, mundane details of being alive in the modern world. But a few more habits continue to haunt me.

◆ I can't stand eating in conference rooms. Really, eating in offices ever. I am all for sitting down at a real lunch. Even (shock!) having a glass of wine.

◆ When people say, "Who are you to judge?" Well, when it comes to behavior, judgment is about taste and values. A person who makes no judgments has no distinct politics or view of the world. Sometimes we deserve to be judged and even sometimes we deserve to be judged poorly. That's how we learn and become better people.

◆ If the bill comes and you ordered a porterhouse while your friend ordered a salad then pay more. In fact, just take care of the bill. In another situation that may be more complicated, offer to leave the tip. On the flip side, don't go through itemizing the bill like an accountant. Just divvy it up and pay your share (even if it's a little more than your share). One friend who takes a lot of people to dinner just gets up from the table and settles the tab. He doesn't make a lot of fanfare about it, just does it quietly, and it's very, very elegant.

GRIEVANCES
This Is Killing Me

"Never ever, under no circumstances, even if your dentist tells you to, should a gentleman spit. But if you must, make sure no one is around." —**Christopher DeLorenzo**

"Public spitting. Completely unacceptable." —**Natty Adams**

"An inability to discuss things calmly." —**Nima Abbasi**

"Swearing. There's plenty of mileage to get out of a well-placed *fuck*, but cheap and frequent use of expletives completely devalue its currency. It's easy, and everyone can do it."
—**Miles Fisher**

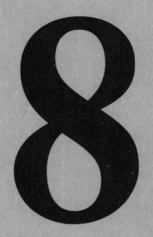

Gray Area

QUESTIONS
FATHERLY ADVICE
SECULAR WISDOM

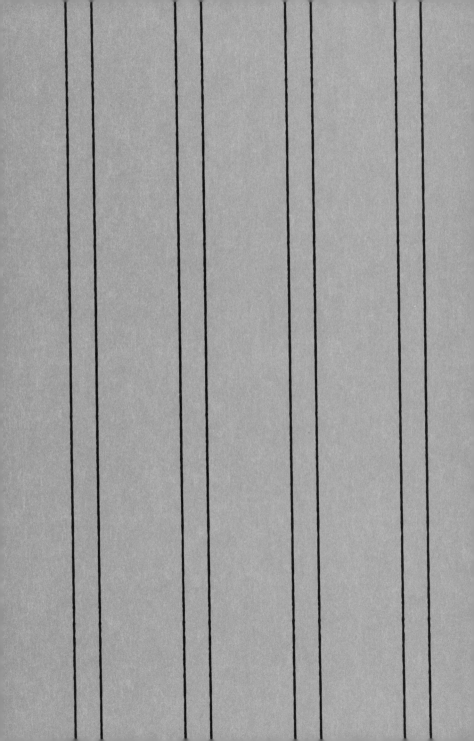

QUESTIONS
Some Answers

"Standing up when a woman leaves the table, enters a room. Outside of period-piece films, I rarely ever see men do this, but then it happens, I think, 'Wait, is this still important? And how have I not been doing this my entire life?'" —Jonathan Baker

I personally stand when it's a nice restaurant. It's an old-fashioned habit I still enjoy. —DC

"Silence—how do you learn the art of silence, the art of being with someone without feeling the need to talk to them?" —Massimo Alba

I think you're speaking about trust. If you can make it through the first minute, then it gets more comfortable. That's largely because there is an understanding between you and your friend.

"I prefer to cut my food with the knife in my right hand. Can we still be friends?" —Jeremy Kirkland

Nothing to be ashamed of, and perfectly acceptable. We remain friends. Let's do lunch.

"What is the maximum number of guests one is allowed to bring to a pool party?" —Ben Greenberg

More than one guest is always pushing it, unless you consult the host in advance. This is a good problem to have and not one that exists in New York.

"Does 'no gift' really ever mean 'no gift'?"
—Ben Greenberg

Send a gift in advance (if it's a milestone, like a major birth-day, and it seems warranted). If it's a party in somebody's home, a bottle of champagne is always welcome.

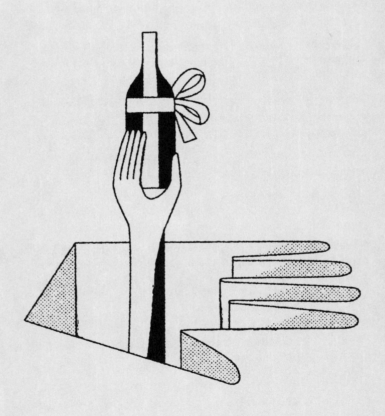

"Wearing belts—I don't understand the point if your pants fit well. Without fail I will be ridiculed at a family party or gathering by a cousin or uncle whose pants look more like drapery than apparel." —Edge Trullinger

I too am belt-agnostic. I like very functional army belts in khaki or blue canvas with metal buckles when wearing chinos (cost: minimal). Or fancy skin belts with O-loops when wearing gray flannels or corduroys (cost: embarrassing).

"I was taught always to open the door for a woman, but it's a tough time for chivalry. Do I open the door for her or not?" —Curt Benham

I definitely hold it—unless it's a revolving door, in which case you can enter first. You ideally hold a cab door, but sometimes there's traffic and you're in a rush and other times a woman is wearing a dress and doesn't feel like sliding across the vinyl seat. I take the plunge and go first. This is New York, after all.

"What is the best response when someone you really like and respect has invited themselves to a private event to which you are not allowed to bring guests? Better yet, you are allowed to bring guests, but you know the host vehemently dislikes the person who has just invited themselves to the event." —Ben Greenberg

Tricky. I think honesty is best here. "I can't bring anybody to the party, I'm sorry." And propose another time to get together very soon. This brief awkward conversation is better than an entire awkward evening.

"There's a gray area these days around smartphones. As soon as someone engages a phone, they are no longer actively present, no longer sincere and engaged with you directly. When it comes to the courtesy of attention, how is the presence of a smartphone politely resolved?" —Miles Fisher

This is tough. When one person takes their phone out then other people at the table usually do as well. I try not to do this and just wait for the other person to stop and they usually do it more quickly if you're making it clear that you're waiting for them. Nothing worse than seeing a table of six people all looking at their phones.

"Tipping on everything aside from restaurants. What do you tip your housekeeper? What do you tip a delivery person? What sort of holiday gift are you supposed to give your dry cleaner? Do you have to tip everyone you deal with at a hotel?" —Jacob Gallagher

Well, this is the big one. I tip my housekeeper a little more than what I pay her for one session, at least $100. For a delivery person, I think about how far they came and how bad the weather is. Usually $5. Dry cleaner? Wow, I'm not that intimate with them. But not a bad idea.

Hotels are interesting. For me, it has to do with how nice it is, how long I was there and how much I used their services (the concierge) and if I felt close to them. I leave money for the maid—usually $10, or $20 for a suite or series of rooms. And money for the concierge (though not in Japan), usually $20, that I hand to him in an envelope. Doorman at the end of stay, $5 or $10, again depending on how much they helped me.

"I've always wondered if I should adopt my own vernacular or a more euphemistic form when discussing the death of someone else's friend or loved one. I personally have always cringed at euphemisms in general. Using softening language for an ugly or unfortunate reality of life does not, in fact, soften the reality, and at a larger level, I think we're all healthier adults if we learn to acknowledge the unfortunate inevitabilities of life rather than attempt to bury them in the saccharine language of a Hallmark greeting card. I'm always very simple and candid when describing the painful deaths of people I am close to. My father *died*. My brother *died*. My grandparents *died*. None of them 'passed.' I'm happy to suspend my standards. In certain circumstances, even the most obvious rules of effective communication are made to be broken." —Alex Williams

I feel the same way. I prefer direct language. But it's hard, especially if the person who's suffering hasn't started to use it yet. So in other words, Alex: I feel the pain of your loss.

FATHERLY ADVICE
World Wise

"As a transplant from France, there are some US habits that I'm still getting used to, after more than fifteen years here. The main one is the general lack of proper greetings. In France, we shake hands every day, or we kiss on the cheeks. Every day, not just when we meet someone for the first time.

"But what really drives me crazy is when the New York pace gets in the way of basic gallantry. Men rushing and pushing women out of the subway car, not even thinking of holding a door, rushing to grab that bus seat before that woman gets it. It is almost an everyday occurrence and it still boils my blood!" —**Greg Lellouche**

"The essence of being a gentleman, even in this sneakers-and-hoodies era, is knowing how to take a compliment. There is nothing more annoying than giving someone a nugget of sincere praise and having them feel obliged out of a misplaced sense of 'manners' to deny the compliment with false humility—'no, really, that Pulitzer/Olympic gold medal/admission to Harvard Law/sleepover date with Scarlett Johansson was just a silly little thing . . . don't know how I ended up with one.' It's hard to give a compliment, especially a sincere one. In many cases, you're saying something about another person that you really would rather have people saying about yourself. So as the compliment giver, the last thing you want to do, once you've swallowed your own envy enough to dial up a shout-out, is to get into an argument about whether the subject will in fact accept the gift or end up

in an argument about whether he or she deserves it. To deny
a compliment is actually a bit of a dis to the compliment giver,
because it subtly calls into question the judgment and/or taste
level of the giver. If you recognize that someone looks amazing
in a $5,000 bespoke suit from Savile Row, the last thing you
want to hear is, 'Oh, no, this old thing? It's nothing, really.'
As the recipient, you should know that the giver knows that
you spent $5,000 for that very reaction, and the giver likely
doesn't have $5,000 of his own to elicit the same response
from others. So if you're the recipient, just be honest. Smile
and give a sincere thanks in return, which acknowledges the
obvious: You worked very hard to earn that compliment, so
you are grateful that someone took the time to give it."
—**Alex Williams**

"My favorite bit of social advice my dad ever gave me was to
know when an argument wasn't worth it. Or, as he put it:
'Sometimes you have to choose between being right and being
happy.' I'm fairly certain this was specifically meant as a warning about arguing with the women you love." —**Natty Adams**

"My dad always dropped the passengers in his car as close to
the front door of the restaurant or theater as possible, then
he headed off solo to find a parking space. This was meant
to be advantageous for well-dressed riders. At the end of the
evening, he would bring the car 'around' to the place most
convenient for the group. I enjoyed joining him on this task to
have one-on-one time with my father." —**Dewey Nicks**

"My father taught me bad manners are a form of selfishness—
I'll greet you at the door when you visit, I'll walk you to the
door when you leave. That's how we make contact with other

people, how we share our lives—and how we feel less alone. I've come to realize that manners begin when we figure out that we're not alone in this world." —**Massimo Alba**

"All that's inside *Tiffany's Table Manners* I've found suits me well enough. But one: Do put your elbows on the table. Get close. Converse. Let it be known you want to be there. Two: Take the last bite. Get rid of that distraction. It's just sitting there otherwise, taking folks from the wine that needs to be drunk, the conversation that needs to be had. Three: Don't ever suggest to a fellow diner that they remind you of someone else. At best, she won't know who you're thinking of. More often, she won't take it well." —**Michael Strout**

"Open the door for people. And not just for your better half, but colleagues, friends, strangers, children, pets. There's a kindness in that simple gesture that transcends."
—**Jonathan Baker**

SECULAR WISDOM

Pastor Curt Benham

I met Curt at Sid Mashburn, where he was the extremely well-dressed elder statesman of the Atlanta HQ (but not *too* elder). We felt an affinity right away—he drove an old Mercedes wagon, loves to fly-fish and has a place in his heart for a good tweed jacket. He is also a pastor, and when I asked him for some thoughts about the world today, he gave me what he called his bonus list. He didn't expect it to be published, but it's too good not to. —DC

- Never chew gum in a place where you wouldn't smoke.

- "Black tie optional" means black tie.

- No one has ever regretted being slightly overdressed.

- Never be late, but know when it's good to be not-too-on-time.

- Never wear sandals where you wouldn't take off your shirt.

- Assume that everyone is dealing with some sort of anxiety, so always lean toward mercy.

- Call your mother every Sunday.

CONTRIBUTORS

Nima Abbasi is the founder of Kaboom Ventures. He lives in New York.

Nathaniel "Natty" Adams is a writer. His most recent book is *We Are Dandy*. He lives in Jersey City and Baltimore.

Massimo Alba is the creative director of his own clothing line. He lives in Milan.

Jonathan Baker is the director of marketing for Sid Mashburn. He also covers the Masters Tournament every April. He lives in Atlanta.

Curt Benham is an Anglican priest who also works at Sid Mashburn. He lives in Atlanta.

Chris Benz is the creative director of Bill Blass. He lives in Brooklyn.

Jon Birger is a journalist and the author of *Date-onomics: How Dating Became a Lopsided Numbers Game*. He lives in New York.

Chris Black is the founder of Done to Death Projects and a host of the podcast Public Announcement. He lives in the East Village.

Christopher DeLorenzo is a graphic artist who made all the drawings in this book. He lives in Boston.

Hugues de Pins is a French businessman who has worked at Cartier and Vacheron Constantin. He now lives in New York.

Miles Fisher is an actor and the founder of Cups Coffee. He lives in Los Angeles.

Jacob Gallagher is the men's fashion editor at Off Duty and the author of the "On Trend" column for the *Wall Street Journal*. He lives in Brooklyn.

Dobby Gibson is a poet and the author of four books including the forthcoming *Little Glass Planet* (Graywolf Press, 2019). He lives in St. Paul, Minnesota.

Ben Greenberg is a copywriter. He is on the board of directors of the Mercantile Library. He lives in Cincinnati.

Ted Harrington is the president of Terrapin Stationers. He lives in Stamford, Connecticut.

Tony King is the CEO and creative director of the creative and technology agency King & Partners. Born in London, he lives in New York.

Jeremy Kirkland is the host of the Blamo! podcast. He lives in New York.

Javas Lehn is the founder of the creative agency Javas Lehn Studio. He lives in New York.

Greg Lellouche is the founder of online menswear store No Man Walks Alone. He was born in Paris and lives in New York.

Michael Maccari is the creative director of Perry Ellis. He lives in New York.

Jim Meehan is a bartender and the author of *Meehan's Bartender Manual* and *The PDT Cocktail Book*. He lives in Portland, Oregon.

Kirk Miller is the founder of the tailor Miller's Oath. He lives in Santa Barbara and New York.

Chris Mitchell is a media executive at Condé Nast. He lives with his wife and two sons in Brooklyn.

Matteo Mobilio is a photographer who recently graduated from Brown. He lives in Brooklyn.

Dewey Nicks is a photographer and director. He lives in Carpinteria, California.

Olof Nithenius is a freelance style editor. He also sells his own line of pocket squares. He lives in Gothenburg, Sweden.

Brooks Reitz is the owner of Leon's Oyster Shop, Little Jack's Tavern and Melfi's, and the founder of Jack Rudy Cocktail Co. He lives in Charleston.

Nick Roberts is a senior account executive at Paul+Williams. He lives in New York.

Mark Rozzo is a writer, musician and contributing editor at *Vanity Fair*. He lives in Brooklyn.

Todd Snyder is the creative director of his own clothing line. He lives in New York.

Matt Stiles is the senior director of merchandising at Polo menswear. He lives in New York.

Michael Strout is the cofounder and CEO of the shoe company Founders. He lives in New York.

Ty Tashiro is a psychologist and the author of *AWKWARD: The Science of Why We're Socially Awkward and Why That's Awesome*. He lives in New York City.

Edge Trullinger works at the Sydell Group. He lives in New York.

Alex Williams is a writer for the *New York Times*. He lives in Brooklyn.

ACKNOWLEDGMENTS

Some writers retreat to the woods and emerge from isolation with a long manuscript and an even longer beard. I am not one of those writers. This book is the result of the insight and talent of many, a true collaboration with people I admire.

I'd like to thank the funny and wise contributors for sharing their savvy opinions; Christopher DeLorenzo for his brilliant illustrations that set the tone for this book; my editor Rebecca Kaplan, creative director John Gall and everybody at Abrams for their vision, expertise and support; my agent and consigliere, Stephanie Koven, who keeps me on the path with the right balance of warmth and discipline; my close friends who set an example by leading generous and interesting lives.

Finally, I'd like to thank my parents, David and Wendy, and my sister, Sarah, whose sense of style, humor and (yes!) manners make their company a basic pleasure of my life.

Salut!

ABOUT THE AUTHOR

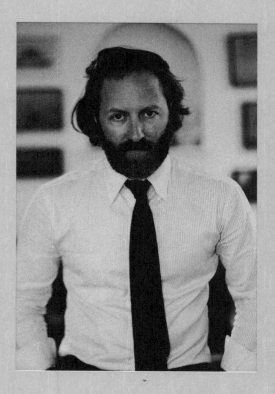

David Coggins is the author of the *New York Times* best-seller *Men and Style*. He has written about style, art, design, travel, drinking, fly-fishing and manners for numerous publications, including *Esquire*, the *Financial Times*, the *Wall Street Journal*, *Art in America* and *Robb Report*. He is a contributing editor of *Condé Nast Traveler*. He lives in New York.

Editor: Rebecca Kaplan
Designer: John Gall
Co-Designer: Najeebah Al-Ghadban
Production Manager: Anet Sirna-Bruder

Library of Congress Control Number: 2017949401

ISBN: 978-1-4197-2733-7
eISBN: 978-1-68335-231-0

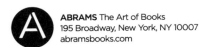
ABRAMS The Art of Books
195 Broadway, New York, NY 10007
abramsbooks.com